VIRTUAL HUMAN-ANIMAL INTERACTIONS

Interest in the field of human-animal interactions is burgeoning, and researchers and educators are keen to understand the science undergirding research that helps us understand interactions between people and animals. Recently, exciting and innovative research is focusing on how people's virtual interactions with animals can enhance their learning, social interactions, and well-being. This research aims to answer questions such as, "What types of interactions do people have with animals in a virtual context? How do people access and experience their virtual interactions with animals? Do virtual interactions with animals hold potential to enhance people's well-being and learning in the same way that in-person interactions with animals have been documented? What educational strategies could be employed to enhance people's virtual interactions with animals? How can we respect animals as research participants within a virtual context?" Drawing from seminal and cutting-edge research in the field of human-animal interactions, these questions and others are answered in *Virtual Human-Animal Interactions*. Research-informed and grounded in critical discussions of theory and practice, this book challenges readers to reconceptualize their understanding of research and practice exploring the complexities inherent in, and arising from, people's virtual interactions with animals. Further, with an eye to the future, this book illuminates readers' thinking around the empirical and practical implications of facilitating interactions between people and animals within virtual contexts. Researchers and educators from across disciplines will find *Virtual Human-Animal Interactions* both scientifically savvy and practical.

Christine Yvette Tardif-Williams, PhD, is an associate professor in the Department of Child and Youth Studies in the Faculty of Social Sciences at Brock University. Dr. Tardif-Williams is grateful to work, live, and cultivate knowledge on the traditional territory of the Haudenosaunee and Anishinaabe peoples.

John-Tyler Binfet, PhD, is an associate professor in the Okanagan School of Education at the University of British Columbia, where he is the director of the *Building Academic Retention through K9s* program (B.A.R.K.). Dr. Binfet is grateful to work, live, and cultivate knowledge on the traditional territory of the Syilx Okanagan peoples.

Virtual Human-Animal Interactions

Supporting Learning, Social Connections
and Well-Being

**Christine Yvette Tardif-Williams and
John-Tyler Binfet**

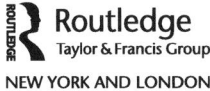

NEW YORK AND LONDON

First published 2023
by Routledge
605 Third Avenue, New York, NY 10158

and by Routledge
4 Park Square, Milton Park, Abingdon, Oxon, OX14 4RN

Routledge is an imprint of the Taylor & Francis Group, an informa business

ISBN: 9781032358024 (hbk)
ISBN: 9781032356419 (pbk)
ISBN: 9781003327868 (ebk)

DOI: 10.4324/9781003327868

Typeset in Times New Roman
by Apex CoVantage, LLC

Funding: This project was made possible, in part, to funding from the *Social Sciences and
Humanities Research Council of Canada* (#435–2021–0678) awarded to both authors.

Dedication

Dedicated to the memory of my mother who inspired in me an affinity for all animals and taught me to look deeply into an animal's eyes to behold their unconditional love, tenderness, and wisdom.
Christine Yvette Tardif-Williams

This book is dedicated to the volunteer handlers, therapy dogs, research assistants, students, and staff of the University of British Columbia's *Building Academic Retention through K9s* (B.A.R.K.) program. It was my intention to honor their hard work throughout this book.
John-Tyler Binfet

Contents

Figures

Tables

Meet the Authors

Christine Yvette Tardif-Williams

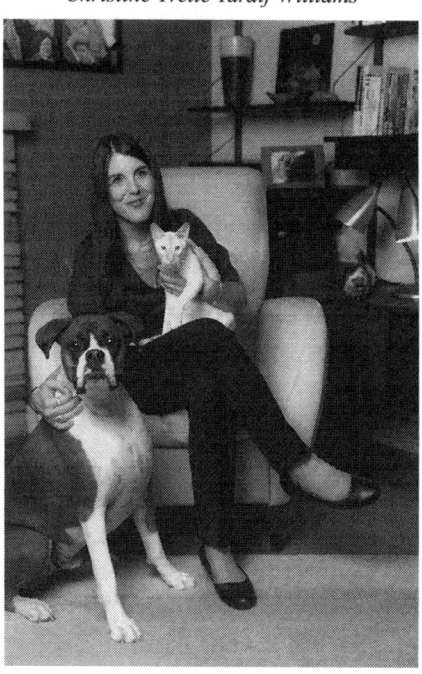

Source: Adam CK Vollick Photography

Christine Yvette Tardif-Williams is an associate professor in the Department of Child and Youth Studies at Brock University and has taught in the postsecondary context for 20 years. Dr. Tardif-Williams's research adopts basic and applied approaches and is informed by the interdisciplinary fields of child and youth development and human-animal interactions. Dr. Tardif-Williams has two research streams that focus more broadly on how close bonds within interpersonal and animal relationships shape the social and emotional lives of children and youth. Specifically, Dr. Tardif-Williams's research examines human-animal interactions, children's relationships with animals, child maltreatment, parent-child attachment, and communication and conflict. Dr. Tardif-Williams's research on children's and dog handlers' experiences with animals and therapy dogs in a variety of learning contexts has been published in *Anthrozoös*, *Society and Animals*, the *Human-Animal Interaction Bulletin*, *Pet Behavior Science,* and *Psychology of Language and Communication*.

John-Tyler Binfet

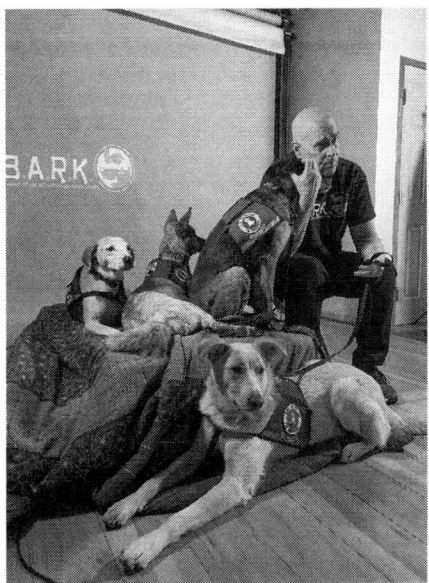

Source: F. L. L. Green Photography

John-Tyler Binfet is an associate professor in the Faculty of Education at the University of British Columbia, Okanagan campus. His research explores prosocial behaviour in children and adolescents and the effects of canine-assisted interventions on college student well-being. Dr. Binfet is the author of two previous books including the recently published *Cultivating Kindness: An Educator's Guide* (2022; University of Toronto Press) and a coauthor of *Canine-Assisted Interventions: A Comprehensive Guide to Credentialing Therapy Dog Teams* (Binfet & Hartwig, 2020; Routledge). His research on the effects of canine-assisted interventions has been published in *Anthrozoös*, the *Journal of Mental Health*, and the *Journal of Veterinary Behavior* among elsewhere. Dr. Binfet is the founder and director of UBC's *Building Academic Retention through K9s* (B.A.R.K.) program that was established in 2012 and routinely sees 60+ therapy dogs and their handlers participate in on-campus and community programming.

1 Introduction

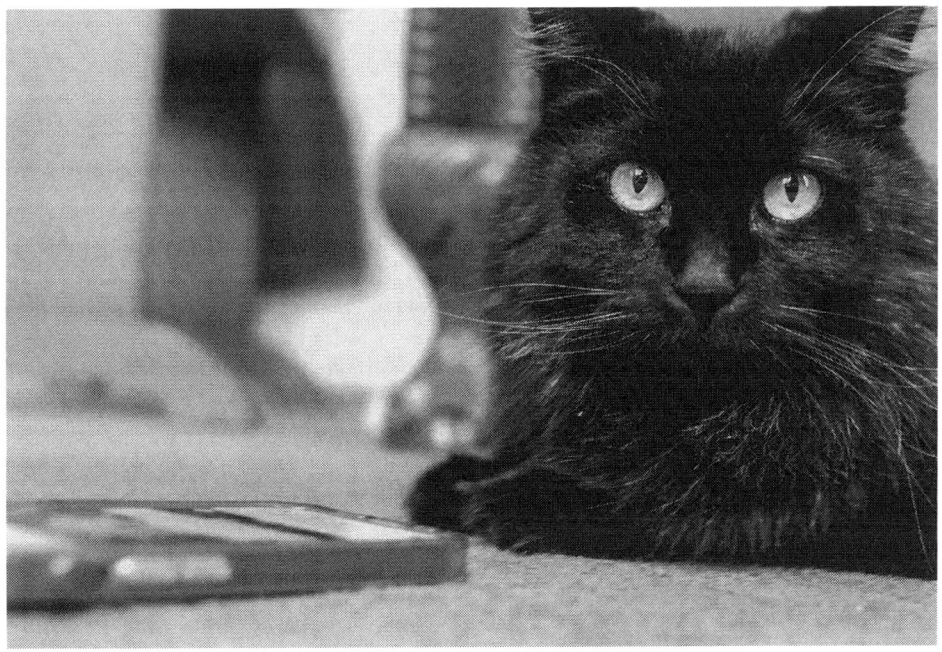

Figure 1.1 Buddy, a black cat, gazing into the camera frame with a cell phone lying nearby

Source: F. L. L. Green Photography

Scenario

Please mom! I really want a kitten, why can't we get one?

Megan has been pleading with her mom for several months to get a kitten. Megan knows in her heart that they can't get a kitten because her younger sister, Amanda, is allergic to cats. Still, she tries to convince her mom that she'd be responsible and feed and groom the kitten every day and that she'd keep the kitten in her room. Megan's mom explains that this will not work and briefly considers getting a family dog, but she knows that she doesn't have the time or finances to care for a puppy now that she is a newly single parent and has started a new job. Since her parents' divorce, Megan has been feeling sad, and

DOI: 10.4324/9781003327868-1

she has grown quiet with her sister at home and with her peers at school. Desperate to fulfill her daughter's social and emotional need for a companion animal, Megan's mom wonders about a virtual companion animal. She's recently heard in the news about online companion animals and how some children develop meaningful connections with them, like the bonds they develop with live animals. She wonders if spending time with a kitten online would help Megan feel better and enjoy hanging out with her sister and friends once again.

Questions for Reflection

1. What types of animals could Megan engage with virtually?
2. In what ways could Megan engage with animals in a virtual context?
3. Could Megan engage in sustained and meaningful interactions with animals virtually?
4. Could Megan develop emotional attachments to animals in a virtual context?

Overarching Aims of the Book

Humans' interactions with animals are long-standing, complex, intricately interwoven, and defined by mutual affinity. History is replete with stories and images of animals performing feats of heroism, engaging in grand adventures, and quietly sharing their lives with humans. Further, there is a growing body of empirical research focused on the intricacies of humans' in-person interactions with animals. This book embraces current technological advances and extends the focus on humans' interactions with animals to include the virtual context. In this book, we welcome advances in technology as an invitation to charter new territory exploring humans' interactions with animals. But what kinds of interactions do people have with animals in a virtual context and how do people experience their virtual interactions with animals? This book explores this exciting and innovative area of study and holds the potential to inspire educators, school and camp counsellors, and researchers working with diverse learners. Our aim in writing this book is to offer a research-informed guide with practical applications for researchers, educators, and practitioners interested in harnessing the potential of virtual interactions to support people's learning, social connections, and well-being. This book begins with an arm's-length overview of the field of human-animal interactions (HAI) and the subsidiary fields of the human-animal bond (HAB) and animal-assisted interventions (AAIs), followed by an empirically grounded exploration of the varied pathways and content available for virtually interacting with animals and provides readers with an overview of the benefits arising from these experiences.

Interest in the field of HAI is burgeoning, and researchers, educators, and practitioners are keen to understand the science undergirding research that helps us comprehend the nature and mechanisms fuelling the quality of interactions between people and animals. Recently, exciting and innovative research is focusing on how people's virtual interactions with animals are built upon and extend in-person interactions and how they might also enhance people's learning, social interactions, and well-being. Drawing on current empirical research, this book explores the following questions:

- In what ways do people virtually interact with animals?
- Do virtual interactions with animals hold potential to enhance people's learning, social connections, and well-being in the same way that in-person interactions with animals have been documented to do?

Table 1.1 Commonly Used Acronyms Found Throughout Our Book

Acronym	Definition
HAI	Human-Animal Interactions
HAB	Human-Animal Bond
AAI	Animal-Assisted Interventions
CAI	Canine-Assisted Interventions
EAI	Equine-Assisted Interventions
VHAI	Virtual Human-Animal Interactions
AAT	Animal-Assisted Therapy
AAE/P	Animal-Assisted Education/Pedagogy
AAC	Animal-Assisted Coaching
AAA	Animal-Assisted Activities

- What educational strategies could be employed to enhance people's virtual interactions with animals?
- How can we respect animals as research participants within a virtual context?

In each chapter of this book, we delve deeper into these exciting questions. We draw on seminal and cutting-edge research conducted with diverse groups to help answer these questions and excavate the landscape of people's emotional and social experiences with animals in a virtual context. Further, we suggest ways in which readers can redesign and reconsider their understanding of research and practice exploring the complexities inherent in, and arising from, people's virtual interactions with animals. We offer our book as a useful resource for anyone interested in learning more about the empirical and practical implications of facilitating interactions between people and animals within virtual contexts, equipping readers to both be critical consumers of virtual HAIs and to craft their own virtual HAI opportunities and experiences.

In this introductory chapter, we introduce readers to the field of HAI including the study of virtual human-animal interactions (VHAIs) and we define key terminology (see Table 1.1 for a list of acronyms used throughout the book). We also outline the major theoretical frameworks undergirding HAIs and discuss how these inform this book's focus on VHAIs. We explicitly establish links between VHAIs and issues of equity, diversity, inclusion, and Indigeneity. We conclude with an overview of the book chapters.

Introduction to Key Terminology

Defining Human-Animal Interactions

We begin by defining several key terms relevant to our consideration of VHAIs. First, we note that HAI represents a broad umbrella term that includes several subfields. We recognize there are different interpretations of just how HAI, HAB, and AAI are interconnected (e.g., see recent interpretations by Fine & Chastain Griffin, 2022 and Parbery-Clark et al., 2021) and offer a model explicating how these terms are positioned relative to one another as we nest VHAIs within the broader HAI field (see Figure 1.2).

HAI is a growing field of research and practice and involves the study of how humans relate to and emotionally, psychologically, and physically interact with animals. Broadly, research on HAI is focused on the reciprocal and interactive relations between humans and animals

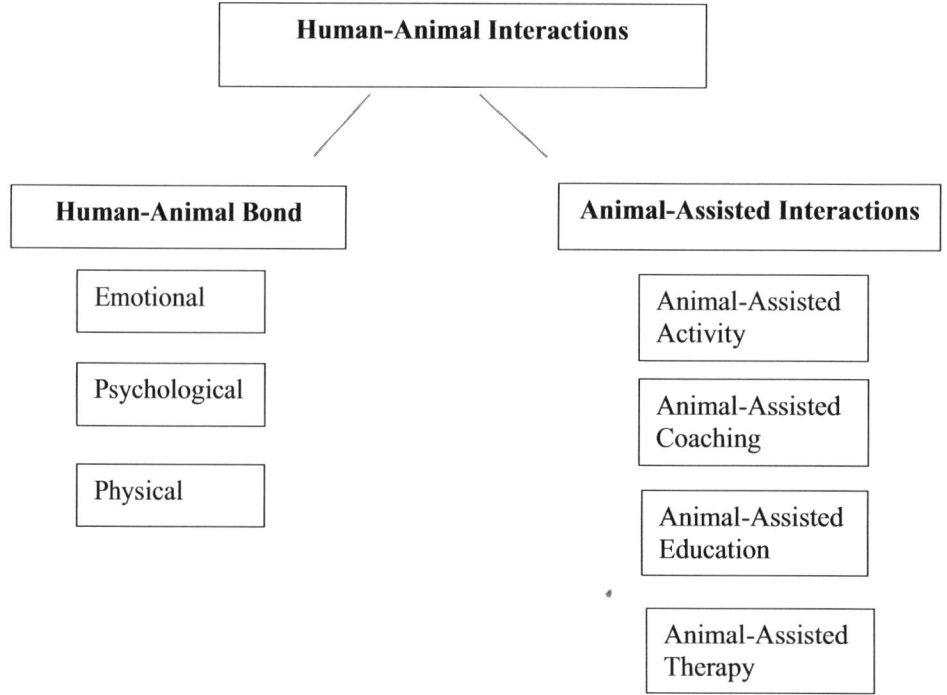

Figure 1.2 Types of human-animal interaction research and practice

(Amiot & Bastian, 2015). It is worth noting that, increasingly, people are sharing their lives with animals. Currently, close to 70% of North American families share their homes and lives with at least one companion animal, which often is a dog or cat (American Pet Products Association, 2022; McElwain, 2020), and, globally, we observed an increased interest in companion animal adoption, particularly for dogs, following the Covid-19 pandemic (Ho et al., 2021). Research in the field of HAI aims to understand the nuances of what motivates people to spend time with animals and to illuminate the varied learning, social, and well-being impacts for both people and animals. To date, a substantial body of research has examined the benefits for people of owning a companion animal and/or interacting with animals such as zoo and farm animals and therapy animals including dogs, cats, horses, and rabbits. In Chapter 2, we'll discuss some of the research findings highlighting the learning, social, and well-being benefits for people over the life course when they spend time with different types of animals and within different contexts (e.g., family- or school-based settings, within the context of AAIs).

Defining the Human-Animal Bond

Next, we note that the HAB is one subfield of HAI research. Research on the HAB is guided by the hypothesis that "the human-animal bond is a mutually beneficial and dynamic relationship between people and animals that is influenced by behaviours essential to the health and wellbeing of both" (American Veterinary Medical Association, 1998, p. 1675). Research on the HAB examines the social attachments that humans develop with nonhuman animals and the ways that the HAB can promote the physiological, psychological, and emotional well-being of both humans and nonhuman animals (for a review of the health benefits of the HAB for humans, see Fine & Ferrell, 2021).

Defining Animal-Assisted Interventions

Another subfield of HAI research involves a focus on AAI. Here, it is important to note that although there is some obvious overlap, the HAB and AAI are distinct research subfields falling under the broader umbrella of HAI. Further, research on AAI is characterized by a great deal of definitional variability and includes a spectrum of goal-oriented and therapeutic interventions that incorporate various animal species with the goal of supporting people's learning, social connections, and physical and mental well-being (Howell et al., 2022; Santaniello et al., 2020). As illustrated in Figure 1.2, these interventions include animal-assisted activities (AAA), animal-assisted therapy (AAT), animal-assisted education/pedagogy (AAE/P), and animal-assisted coaching (AAC) (Fine & Ferrell, 2021; Parbery-Clark et al., 2021). Interested readers may want to refer to the definitions for animal-assisted activity and guidelines for safeguarding animal wellness published in a white paper by the International Association for Human-Animal Interaction Organizations (IAHAIO, 2014). AAIs share the premise that spending time with animals is beneficial to people's physical and mental health (Fine & Weaver, 2018) and involve "any intervention that intentionally includes or incorporates animals as part of a therapeutic or ameliorative process or milieu" (Kruger & Serpell, 2006, p. 25). It is important to note, however, that AAT is unique in involving a structured and planned intervention led by a trained mental health practitioner and trained therapy dog (Fine & Ferrell, 2021). Also, it is worth reiterating here that AAIs vary in terms of their structures (i.e., AAT is highly structured, whereas AAC is more flexibly structured); underlying goals, which can be educational, therapeutic, and emotionally supportive in orientation; and type of animal involved, with equine- and canine-assisted interventions (EAI and CAI, respectively) being very popular (for a review, see Parbery-Clark

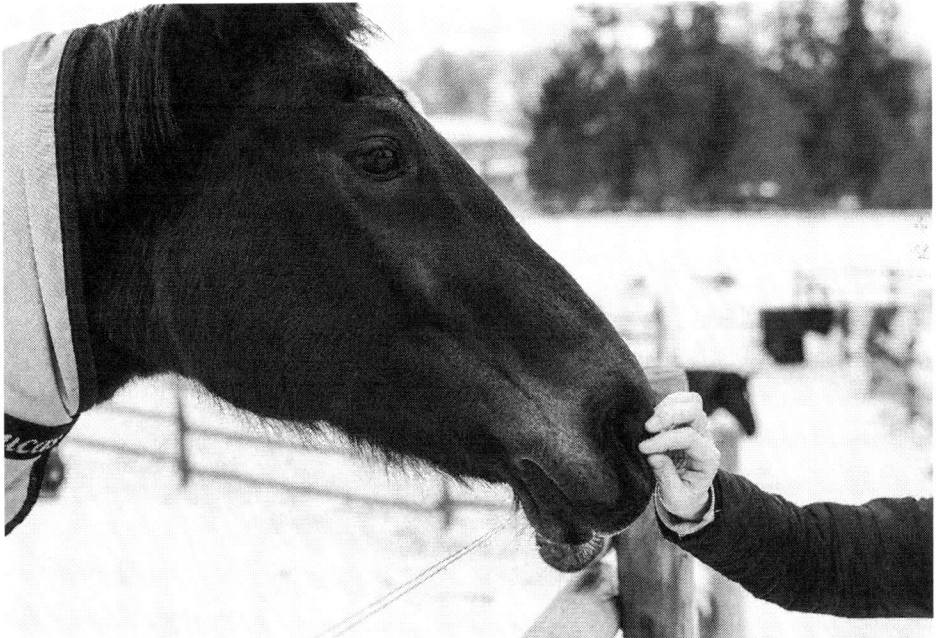

Figure 1.3 Human-horse connection: A horse named Kingston getting his nose rubbed

Source: F. L. L. Green Photography

et al., 2021). While there is an extensive body of research on the effects of equine-assisted activities and therapies on human learning and well-being (as discussed in Chapter 2), there is a preponderance of research involving canines, and we acknowledge our bias in sharing our own canine-centric research findings. However, in the chapters to follow, we are also careful to illustrate the variety of species participating in HAI and AAI research. Last, AAI can take place in a variety of settings, and we argue in this book that the virtual context is one relatively untapped and promising setting.

Defining Canine-Assisted Interventions

Recently, AAIs that involve canines and their human handlers – one category of AAIs – have become increasingly popular across a multitude of contexts (e.g., university and college campuses, elementary schools, medical and dental offices, hospitals, public libraries) to reduce stress and anxiety, boost mood, provide comfort, and support reading and learning (Binfet & Hartwig, 2020). These CAIs or canine visitation (Pendry & Vandagriff, 2019) sessions have been defined as "bringing together of credentialed canine-assisted intervention teams and members of the public in a specified setting with the purpose of enhancing human well-being" (Binfet & Hartwig, 2020, p. 10). Generally, the goals of CAIs or canine visitation sessions include providing comfort, increasing positive affect, reducing stress and anxiety, alleviating loneliness, and facilitating social connections and/or campus connectedness. Of note is that CAIs can be delivered individually or in group settings (including the virtual context) and can involve one or more CAI teams (Binfet & Hartwig, 2020).

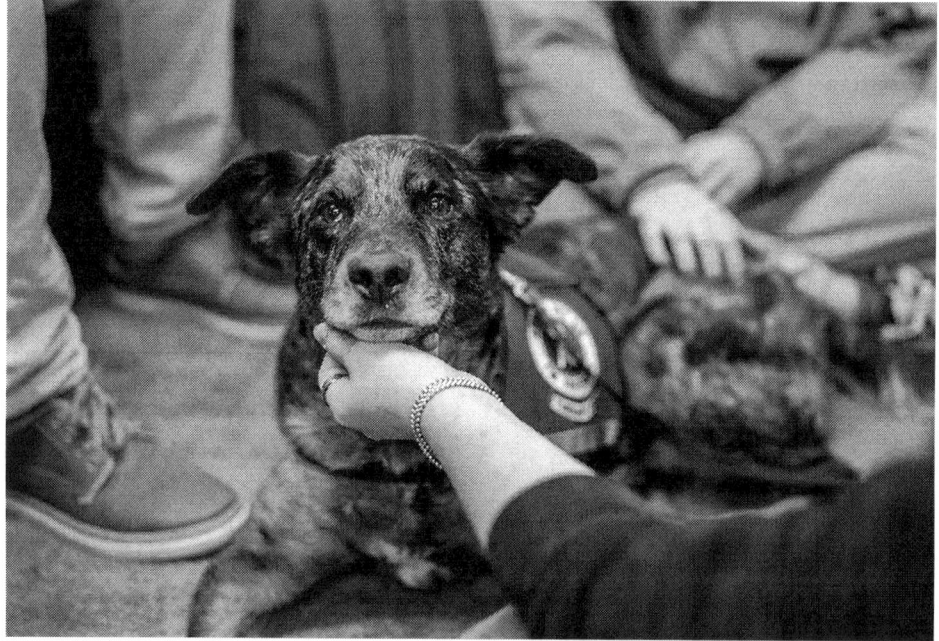

Figure 1.4 Students petting therapy dog Frances from the University of British Columbia's B.A.R.K. program

Source: F. L. L. Green Photography

Clarifying Features of Animal Engagement in Human-Animal Interactions

Moving forward, we need to explore if the noted benefits of in-person HAI apply equally to the virtual context. Notably, in a systematic review of AAIs, Marino (2012) argues that research is needed to examine if involvement of a live animal is necessary for positive therapeutic effects – this remains an important empirical question. We add that further research is required to examine nuances in level and type of animal engagement necessary for positive impacts on people's learning, social connections, and well-being. For example, is it necessary for animals to be in close physical proximity to people or for people to have direct, physical contact with animals? As noted previously, meaningful HAIs unfold in a variety of contexts. In this book, we explore the virtual context as an innovative and exciting new space for HAIs.

What Are Virtual Human-Animal Interactions?

So far, we have discussed interventions involving in-person HAI. To date, and as we discuss further in Chapter 2, research has focused on people's in-person interactions with animals more broadly and how these interactions can either help students learn within school-based contexts or how they can foster healing and emotional resilience among people in more general contexts. In this book, we examine the varied pathways and content elucidating people's virtual interactions with animals (e.g., classroom learning, therapeutic context, social context of sharing pictures and videos of family pets or playing virtual games with animal themes). We seek to illuminate nuances in people's VHAIs. Often, people seek out ways to interact virtually with animals, or people's virtual interactions with animals are designed to mirror as closely as possible the type of interactions that they share with animals in person. In fact, they are often designed to facilitate both social connections and a human-animal relationship, factors theorized to contribute to supporting people's well-being by reducing stress and anxiety and bolstering positive affect. In this book, we define VHAIs as interactions between humans and animals using digital technologies and/or within an online, virtual context. We submit that the virtual context is far from being a lonely space existing in a faraway galaxy! We'll explore the many ways that animals captivate our attention and speak to our hearts and minds from across the screen.

We note that VHAIs can involve both active or passive interactions (synchronous or asynchronous platforms, respectively) and can be brief and short-lived or prolonged and sustained in focus. Further, synchronous interactions unfold in real time with people interacting from different locations during specified times (e.g., Skype or Zoom), whereas asynchronous interactions unfold according to a more relaxed schedule wherein people can interact with one another from different locations but at different times (e.g., self-initiated access to standard content in blogs or predefined viewing of animal-themed videos or live videos with animals). In Chapters 3 and 4 we'll consider how animals are engaged synchronously, such as through sharing animal Instagram accounts and TikTok videos, playing animal-themed video games, engaging in immersive virtual animal field trips complete with a live-cam lookout and volunteering virtually at an animal shelter. As an example, Camille is 12 years old and in seventh grade, and she just launched a *Cat Math Homework Club*. The club consists of several of Camille's classmates and their respective cats, and they meet virtually each Monday evening to cuddle with and share stories about their cats and to work on math assignments. Camille says that having their cats join them helps to keep learning fun and interesting. In this way, the cats offer a calm and comforting presence and are a great social catalyst, which helps to sustain the classmates' homework focus.

We'll then consider how animals are engaged asynchronously such as individually seeking and watching YouTube clips of cute cats and dogs to engaging in digital humane education activities within a classroom or group-based setting. Simone is a 16-year-old high school student who describes herself as very shy and quiet but who loves to regularly post pictures and videos of her two rabbits, Lennox and Frasier, on Instagram. For instance, Simone beams when she describes how many *followers* her rabbits have, and she is quick to share that she met two close school friends through Lennox and Frasier's shared Instagram account. Camille's and Simone's virtual interactions with animals suggest that features of synchronous and asynchronous virtual platforms will appeal to people differently and research is needed that examines the nuances of how, why, and when people virtually engage with animals.

Our Shifting World and Virtual Human-Animal Interactions

This book is timely and relevant to researchers, educators, and practitioners for several reasons. First, our world is fast-changing, and technological innovations are steadily and rapidly transforming our daily lives and the quality of social connections. Technological advancements are shaping the way that we communicate and socially and emotionally connect with meaningful people and beloved animals. Rault (2015) posits that the current digital revolution has drastically changed our social relationships as well as our relationships vis-à-vis animals (e.g., live, robotic, or virtual animal interactions). Notably, we continue to witness a rise in animal-related content and videos online and on various social media platforms. In fact, it appears that humans have an inexhaustible enthusiasm for sharing and viewing online videos of their own and others' cute animals. This book considers some of the factors driving this enthusiasm among diverse people. We'll also explore how these VHAIs might be related to the quality of people's learning, social connections, and well-being.

Second, the recent Covid-19 pandemic has showcased the potential of technology to help people connect with family, friends, and work colleagues during especially challenging times. It is likely that people will continue to harness the potential of technology as they increasingly return to in-person interactions. Relatedly, during the Covid-19 pandemic, 30% of American families adopted a new (and sometimes first) companion animal, including dogs (Insurance Research Council, 2022). Both the Covid-19 pandemic and the shifting nature of our social- and work-related interactions are fueling the proliferation and relevance of exploring the meaning of VHAIs. In this regard, the Covid-19 pandemic represents an opportunity to explore the potential of animals to support people's learning, social connections, and well-being.

Exploring the potential of animals to support people's well-being is critical since current research indicates that the Covid-19 pandemic has been linked to the onset of mental health problems such as depression, post-traumatic stress disorder, and increased symptoms related to anxiety disorders among people, particularly university students (Hamza et al., 2021; Kaparounaki et al., 2020; Tang et al., 2020; Wang & Zhao, 2020). In fact, more generally, we are seeing a dramatic rise in mental health challenges (e.g., depression, anxiety, post-traumatic stress disorder, neurodevelopmental disorders) worldwide among diverse people of all ages (World Health Organization, 2021). Further, mental health resources are often overwhelmed, and many see long waitlists to access services. In Chapters 2 and 3, we'll further explore the role of animals to support people's learning, social connections, and well-being in both in-person and virtual contexts.

Third, we are simultaneously witnessing a push to expand accessibility to learning, social, and mental health resources to reach a variety of people, including those living in geographically remote areas or who have communication and mobility challenges such as vision and hearing impairments. There is also a push to expand accessibility to key mental health resources (e.g., online support groups and tools, directory of local supports) for people who have mental health challenges. This is because such challenges often prevent these people from accessing and benefitting from important well-being supports and meaningful in-person interactions with animals. These mental health difficulties might include post-traumatic stress disorder, social anxiety, neurodevelopmental disorders (e.g., autism spectrum disorder, attention deficit hyper-activity disorder), or other exceptionalities (e.g., phobias of specific animal species, social phobia, agoraphobia). In these situations, rapid developments in technology represent exciting opportunities for researchers and educators who are interested in harnessing the benefits of VHAIs to support people's learning, social connections, and well-being.

Last, the relevance of VHAIs is underscored when we consider how our increasingly fast-paced and technology-driven world is often devoid of contact with nature and animals. In fact, some scholars argue that today, more than ever, young people live in a society that is saturated with technology and social media, and many young people live in urbanized settings. In this way, there is a growing disconnect with each successive generation between people and nature. Kahn and colleagues (2009) refer to this process as *environmental generational amnesia* and boldly suggest that this process could become the central psychological problem of our time. To some extent, the process of *environmental generational amnesia* might explain the dramatic rise in mental health challenges we are currently witnessesing (World Health Organization, 2021). This book considers how VHAIs might support – rather than detract from – a vital reconnection with nature and animals. We hope that educators of all ages will be inspired by the ways that technology might be harnessed to virtually connect learners with nature and animals.

Exploring Virtual Human-Animal Interactions Through the Lens of Equity, Diversity, Inclusion, and Indigeneity

Overall, research suggests that HAIs hold potential to support learning, social connections, and well-being among people of all ages. An unknown piece of the HAI research puzzle is whether these benefits extend to the virtual context – a context wherein HAIs are increasingly unfolding and reimagined. As we noted, recent societal shifts in technology use have fueled an increase in VHAIs and have also left researchers and educators scrambling to pivot their in-person human-animal programs to a virtual context (see Dell et al., 2021 for an illustration of this process). The question remains, "Does the virtual human-animal context afford similar and unique benefits as do in-person HAI programs?" In fact, we believe that VHAIs hold the potential to democratize access to key learning and well-being resources by providing path-ways to reach diverse audiences and featuring specialized content. First, as we will explore further in Chapter 2, VHAIs can offer nonthreatening, self-initiated, high-quality, easily acces-sible, and cost-effective learning, social, and well-being support to a diverse audience of peo-ple. Second, researchers and educators could develop specialized curricula in inclusive and sensitive ways to support diverse groups of people. For instance, specialized curricula could be developed that would appeal directly to diverse audiences including, but not limited to, people who have disabilities and people within BIPOC and two-Spirit, lesbian, gay, bisexual, transgender, queer, intersex, and additional sexually and diverse people (2SLGBTQI+) com-munities. In this way, VHAIs can be designed to reach diverse audiences as previously noted and can explicitly address issues of disparity, diversity, and Indigeneity. Due to the potential for increasing accessibility and offering specialized content, VHAIs can be characterized as facilitating equity and inclusion.

Theoretical Frameworks Undergirding Virtual Human-Animal Interactions

The field of HAIs is characterized by varied perspectives outlining the potential mechanisms involved in supporting the development of positive in-person and VHAIs and their impact on people's learning, social connections, and well-being. In fact, several theoretical and methodological frameworks undergird the field ranging from mainly cross-disciplinary to inherently interdisciplinary in focus. These theoretical frameworks are informed by advances in social, developmental, relational, and evolutionary psychology, biology, critical animal studies, animal studies or posthumanism, and media studies (see Table 1.2). Our book's focus is inherently interdisciplinary and draws predominantly on the *biophilia hypothesis* (Kellert & Wilson, 1993; Wilson, 1984), *social support theory* (Cobb, 1976; Cohen & Wills, 1985; Schaefer et al., 1981), *biopsychosocial theory* (e.g., Gee et al., 2021), the *theory of media equation* (Reeves & Nass, 1996), and research on *motivation, engagement, and learning* (Gee et al., 2017; Wohlfarth et al., 2013).

Here, we briefly acknowledge interdisciplinary frameworks such as animal studies or posthumanism (Haraway, 2008) and critical animal studies (Matsuoka & Sorenson, 2018) that offer new and inspiring ways of thinking about animals and animal-human relationships (for a discussion, see Adams, 2018). Notably, posthumanism and critical animal studies frameworks challenge speciesism and anthropocentrism; they seek to challenge traditional boundaries between humans and animals (Haraway, 2008; Shapiro, 2020). In this way, posthumanism and critical animal studies scholars embrace a deeper *animal turn* (Shapiro, 2020) and a *relational ontology* wherein the relations between humans and animals are mutually constitutive (Haraway, 2008; Shapiro, 2020); they are ordinary *beings-in-encounter* in various worlds or contexts (Haraway, 2008). They also emphasize *intersectionality* between humans and animals. *Intersectionality* refers to how different forms of prejudice, oppression, and marginalization are intricately interwoven and must be addressed by considering their interrelationships (Adams, 2015; Potts, 2010). Further, the field of critical animal studies expressly presents animal liberation as a social justice movement that intersects with other related movements for positive change (i.e., trans-species social justice). Further, critical animal frameworks integrate academic research and political activism and examine societal boundaries between humans and animals, the role of animals in human societies, how animals are represented, and humans' ethical duty toward animals. We consider some of these exciting ideas in the chapters to follow when we discuss current trends and future directions in reimagining HAI in a virtual context (Chapter 3), the unexplored potential of qualitative research methods (Chapter 3), and safeguarding animal welfare in a virtual context (Chapter 5).

Biophilia Hypothesis

Our book draws conceptually on Wilson's (1984) *biophilia hypothesis*, which asserts that people have an "innate tendency to focus on life and lifelike processes" (Wilson, 1984, p. 1). Thus, animals offer a live stimulus, which, as Serpell (1996) describes, serves to draw the interest of the participant, focus or concentrate his or her attention, and has an overall calming effect. The biophilia hypothesis is especially relevant at this historical time when it has been argued that humans (especially when living in urban areas) are experiencing *nature deficit disorder* due to modern practices that often detract from meaningful interactions with nature and animals (Louv, 2008). This can, over successive generations, lead to *environmental generational amnesia* (Kahn et al., 2009). Both the concept of *nature deficit disorder* and *environmental generational amnesia* have been hypothesized to contribute to decreased physical and mental

Table 1.2 Theoretical Frameworks Undergirding Human-Animal Interactions

Theories	Description	Key Resources
Attachment Theory	Humans and animals are biologically predisposed to protect their offspring to ensure their survival. In turn, young children and animals are biologically predisposed to maintain close physical proximity with a sensitive and responsive attachment figure who can offer protection and care, especially during stressful times	• Bowlby, 1969
Biophilia Hypothesis	The natural human instinct to seek connections with other nonhuman forms of life and lifelike processes.	• Kellert & Wilson, 1993 • Wilson, 1984
Biopsychosocial	An interdisciplinary model which proposes that people's interactions with dogs (and animals) may have important impacts on each of the biological, social, and psychological aspects of human health.	• Gee et al., 2021
Posthumanism and Critical Animal Studies	Posthumanism and critical animal studies are interdisciplinary frameworks that challenge speciesism and anthropocentrism; they seek to challenge traditional boundaries between humans and animals. These frameworks embrace a deeper *animal turn* and a *relational ontology* wherein the relations between humans and animals are mutually constitutive.	• Adams, 2015 • Haraway, 2008 • Matsuoka & Sorenson, 2018 • Potts, 2010 • Shapiro, 2020
Developmental Relational Model	The application of relational developmental systems models, which explore bidirectional influences between individuals and their contexts, to the study of HAI across the life course.	• Mueller, 2014
Media Equation Theory	The theory that humans tend to respond to media technologies and media content as if they were real or human. The media provides an interaction, giving it human-like qualities.	• Reeves & Nass, 1996
Motivation, Engagement, and Learning	A unified framework that suggests that animals might impact people's learning and social interactions by increasing motivation and/or self-efficacy. The inclusion of an animal in targeted activities can have an indirect effect on learning by increasing people's motivation and self-efficacy and enhancing engagement/attention and executive functions.	• Gee et al., 2017 • Wohlfarth et al., 2013

(Continued)

Table 1.2 (Continued)

Theories	Description	Key Resources
Social Support Theory	A model which suggests that social relationships, including interactions with animals, can provide a sense of comfort and connectedness and offer a defense against stress and anxiety through various means of support.	• Cobb, 1976 • Cohen & Wills, 1985 • Schaefer et al., 1981

health. Fine and colleagues have argued that people's overwhelming reliance on technology has contributed to people spending less time in nature and with animals or nature deprivation. To some extent, we believe that this is the case. However, we believe that VHAIs offer a promising avenue toward reconnecting people with nature's lessons and rewilding and sensitizing people's hearts toward nature and animals (Bekoff, 2014). As previously noted, this book considers how VHAIs might support – rather than detract from – a vital reconnection with nature and animals. In fact, we suggest that technological advances can be reimagined and recast as promising tools and, perhaps, a key first step toward reengaging a new generation of learners. We hope that educators of all ages will be inspired by the ways that technology might be leveraged to virtually connect learners with nature and animals. Our book is timely given the recent influx in educational efforts to expose young learners to wild and farm animals through media sources, nature activities, and visits to zoos and aquariums. Further, in our increasingly technologically driven world, where learning and instruction may be void of hands-on contact with nature and with a diversity of animals, developing humane literacy in a virtual context represents a first step toward fostering compassion for all animals and to support concerns for biodiversity conservation in a new generation of learners.

Social Support Theory

Our book is also theoretically informed by Cobb's (1976) *social support theory,* which suggests that social relationships provide a buffer against anxiety, depression, and other related illnesses. Social support theory outlines the conditions of social companionship that foster positive health effects (Cobb, 1976; Hupcey, 1998). For example, research indicates that having a social support network including friends, family, and peers is a vital resource that mediates between stress and mental and physical health and can offset academic stress in undergraduate students (Schaefer et al., 1981; Wilks & Spivey, 2010). Although originally theorized about human companionship, the model endorses a social support hypothesis that can be applied to explain the physiological and psychological benefits of interacting with companion animals (Fine & Weaver, 2018; O'Haire, 2010). Within the context of VHAIs, the animal and other people interacting with an animal, including an animal handler, can be perceived as a sort of social resource supporting people, bolstering people's ability to cope, and buffering people from the adverse effects of stress. Besides providing direct social support, animals also act indirectly as social facilitators or "social lubricants" (Guest et al., 2006; Kruger & Serpell, 2006). Animals often facilitate intimate, one-on-one connections and group interactions, factors theorized to contribute to stress reduction – in this way, animals can also serve a protective function. Past research shows that people with animal companions are perceived as happier, friendlier, less threatening, more relaxed, and more desirable as acquaintances or friends, even when they belong to groups that are sometimes stigmatized (e.g., people using assistive mobility aids (Eddy et al., 2001).

We believe that VHAIs, even if brief, can also promote the formation of vital and lasting social connections and help foster social capital.

Biopsychosocial Theory

Our book also draws on biological theories and Gee et al.'s (2021) *biopsychosocial theory*. According to Beck (2014), our relationship with domestic animals is rooted in evolutionary, psychological, and physiological processes. Biologically, humans are attracted to neotenous features in young animals, which include juvenile features such as large eyes, rounded forehead and ears, and shortened muzzle – humans are biologically attuned to making connections with animals (Beck & Katcher, 1996). Further, according to Bowlby's (1969) attachment theory, humans and animals are biologically predisposed to protect their offspring to ensure their survival. In turn, young children and animals are biologically predisposed to maintain close physical proximity with a sensitive and responsive attachment figure who can offer protection and care, especially during stressful times. The attachment figure provides a secure and safe base that enables young children and animals to explore the environment freely and safely – they are protected from potentially dangerous and stressful situations. Importantly, recent research suggests that humans can develop strong attachments to their companion dogs (Payne et al., 2015) and that dogs can also exhibit attachment styles similar to those developed in humans (Thielke & Udell, 2020). Fine (2014) notes that an animal's dependence and attachment to humans is vital to the development and maintenance of the HAB; in this way, the attachment systems of the infant-parent and human-animal dyads are resonant.

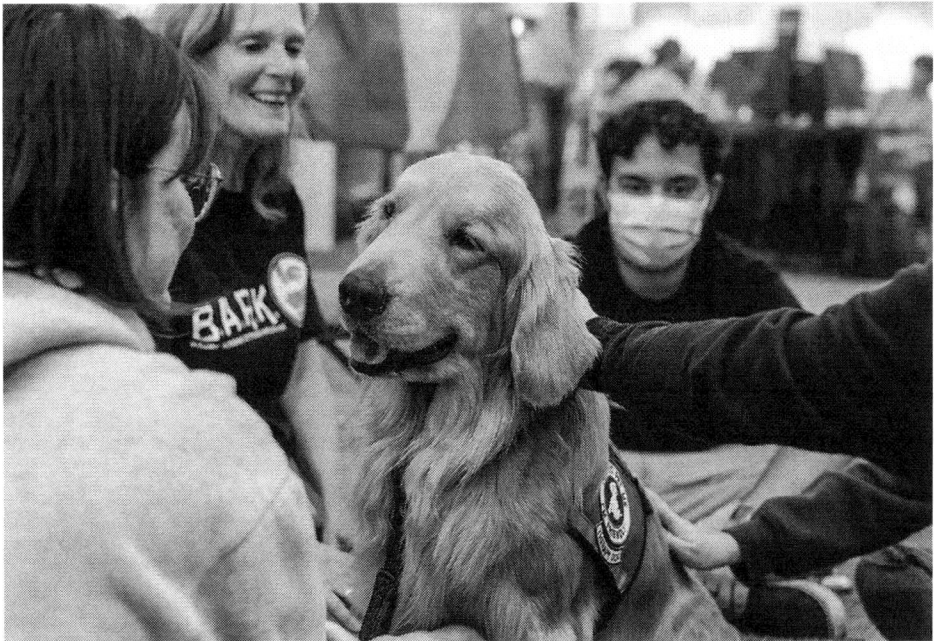

Figure 1.5 University students finding comfort from therapy dog Ember from UBC's B.A.R.K. program

Source: F. L. L. Green Photography

Applying a biopsychosocial approach, Gee et al. (2021) propose that people's interactions with dogs (and other animals) may have important impacts on each of the biological, social, and psychological aspects of human health. Notably, they propose a biological mechanism through which our interactions with a dog can reduce stress and increase positive affect by reducing cortisol levels (a hormone associated with stress) and releasing oxytocin (a hormone associated with attachment and affiliation – the *love* or *bonding* hormone; Rault et al., 2017). Research shows that human-animal bonding is facilitated through interactions involving intimacy and social touching (for a discussion, see Fine & Ferrell, 2021), and recent findings support the stress-buffering benefits for people of interacting with animals (Barker et al., 2016; Handlin et al., 2011; Janssens et al., 2021).

In addition to offering opportunities for direct, social touching, animals can help to create a calm and comforting ambience and provide a sense of visual reassurance, anchoring people in

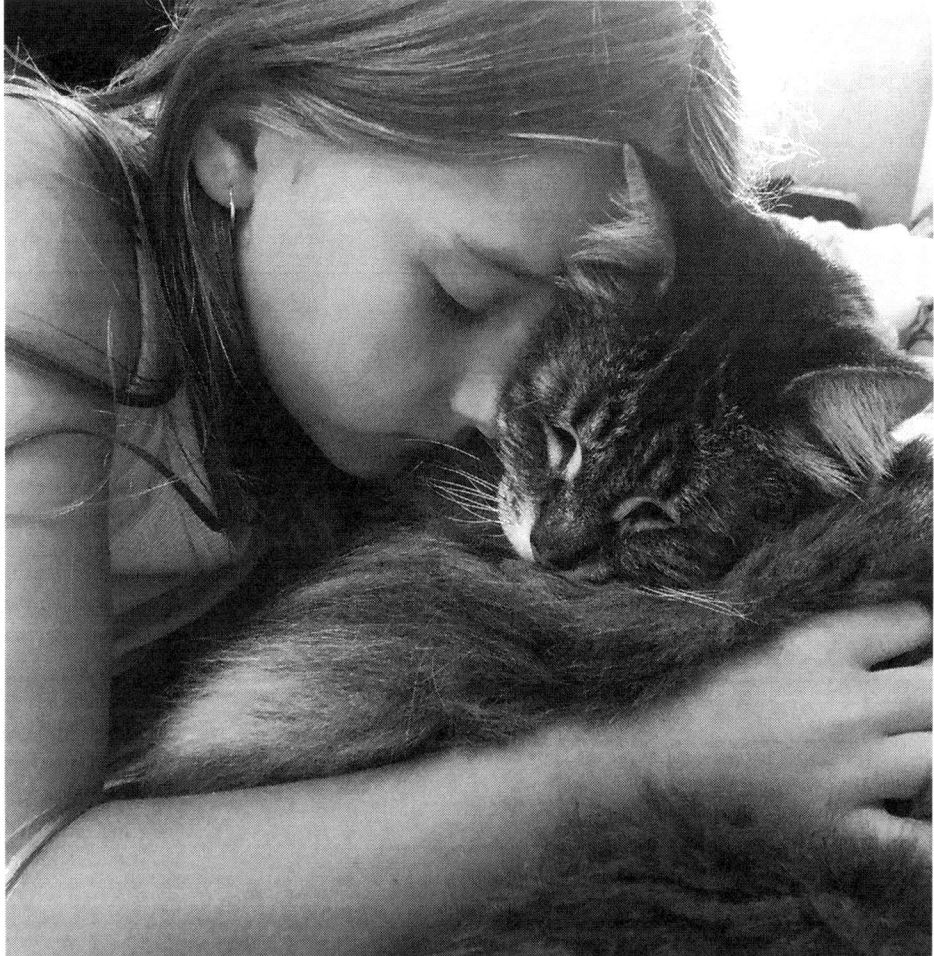

Figure 1.6 A child snuggles with her pet cat

Source: Krista Evans Photography

the present moment. Here, we note that eye gazing plays an important role in communication between humans and animals. In fact, research shows that mutual eye gazing between dogs and their human companions increases oxytocin levels in both dogs and humans – thus promoting a positive oxytocin loop (Nagasawa et al., 2015; Odendaal & Meintjes, 2003). These biological effects may translate to additional positive effects on people's learning and social emotional well-being. Stress and positive affect are two important biological influencers that might further impact learning and social and emotional well-being (Gee et al., 2021). In this way, we submit that VHAIs – which offer opportunities for meaningful mutual human-animal gazing – might have important momentary and longer-lasting impacts on peoples' biological, social, and emotional well-being.

Media Equation Theory

Our book also draws on the *theory of media equation* (Reeves & Nass, 1996) and research on human emotion regulation (Myrick, 2015). According to the theory of media equation, people tend to react to media content in much the same way as they would to real-life interactions, or as if it is happening in real life (Reeves & Nass, 1996). In this regard, researchers have suggested that complex emotional experiences and emotion regulation processes might also extend to our online interactions with animals (Myrick, 2015). Still other researchers have suggested that the virtual context or *telepresence* (i.e., feeling of *being there*) can enhance *social presence* and *flow,* which can, in turn, boost well-being and positive emotions (Zhou et al., 2020). If so, then the positive well-being impacts of HAI might extend to the virtual context. We suggest that VHAIs that offer mediated engagement with animals could offer participants similar *stress-buffering* effects as those found in in-person animal-assisted interventions (e.g., Binfet et al., 2022; Barker et al., 2016; Crossman, 2017; Crossman & Kazdin, 2015; Pendry & Vandagriff, 2019).

Motivation, Engagement, and Learning

Finally, our book draws conceptually on *research related to motivation, engagement, and learning* (Gee et al., 2017; Wohlfarth et al., 2013). One of the ways that animals might impact people's learning, social connections, and well-being is by increasing motivation and/or self-efficacy (Gee et al., 2017). Gee and colleagues (2017) propose a unified framework in which motivation and self-efficacy, engagement/attention and executive functions, self-regulation and stress coping, and social interactions mediate the effect of AAI on learning, social connections, and well-being. The inclusion of an animal in targeted activities can have an indirect effect on learning by increasing people's motivation and self-efficacy and enhancing engagement/attention and executive functions. For instance, canines may increase implicit motives by subconsciously arousing capacities to orient, select, and energize activities such as canine-assisted reading activities (Wohlfarth et al., 2013). Schuck and Fine (2017) suggest that AAIs that include a calm therapy animal can serve to reduce stress and sensory overstimulation in the learning environment and, in this way, help to prime cognitive arousal in learners. They note that these mechanisms can, in turn, elicit greater engagement and motivation and facilitate learning and social skills among children, particularly those who have attention deficit hyperactivity disorder or other learning difficulties. Here, we suggest that in-person and VHAIs equally hold the potential to increase people's motivation to engage in learning and social activities in a sustained way and to increase their feelings of task/social mastery.

Overview of the Book Chapters

We now return to the questions raised at the beginning of this chapter.

- In what ways do people virtually interact with animals?
- Do virtual interactions with animals hold potential to enhance people's learning, social connections, and well-being in the same way that in-person interactions with animals have been documented to do?
- What educational strategies could be employed to enhance people's virtual interactions with animals?
- How can we respect animals as research participants within a virtual context?

Each of these exciting questions is addressed within the chapters that follow. This book begins with a brief overview of HAIs, including VHAIs – an innovative and exciting subdiscipline supported by emerging empirical evidence attesting to its viability as a pathway supporting human well-being. Chapter 2 introduces in-person HAIs as a foundation for VHAIs. We establish that VHAIs constitute a low-barrier, nonthreatening, and easy-to-access resource that, in turn, can foster the pursuit of more formal well-being resources. In addition, we explore the varied iterations of virtual opportunities for HAIs, including the design and delivery of specialized curricula, and consider key social and well-being outcomes arising from virtually connecting with animals. Chapter 3 explores how HAIs are currently being reimagined, recast, and empirically examined within varied virtual contexts. How can we successfully transition in-person AAI to a virtual context to support learners' social and emotional well-being? We draw on parallel research in the field of mental health and provide an overview of the varied ways that virtual mental health support has been successfully offered using both asynchronous and synchronous modes of delivery. We discuss how VHAIs might be more accessible to some people as compared with in-person well-being interventions precisely because they can be accessed at any time of the day and from any location and, in this way, might offer alternative and more timely support when people are experiencing an emotional challenge. Chapter 4 explores the unique role of social media in fostering informal VHAIs. We discuss the different social media platforms that exist and the increasingly important role of social media in people's lives from the Instagram and TikTok trends of younger generations to the popularity of Facebook among adults. We then explore the many ways that animals tend to feature prevalently within social media and discuss some of the ways that informal VHAIs might foster well-being among social media users. Chapter 5 clarifies the importance of animal welfare in a virtual context. This chapter considers how we can create optimal conditions that respect all aspects of animal welfare within virtual contexts. We explore issues of animal consent, working conditions for animals including duration of interactions, and the importance of client education as an aspect of VHAIs. This chapter offers an applied checklist for considering animal welfare within virtual contexts. In Chapter 6, we provide recommendations for best practices for how to optimally design, structure, and deliver VHAIs. We explore the mechanics of structuring VHAIs, including considerations of handler training and preparation, the use of scripts, videography, how to engage virtual viewers, and the assessment of the benefits of interactions on participants. This chapter also provides a checklist for readers, offering them support and guidance in the creation and actualization of VHAIs. Our last chapter, Chapter 7, provides an overview of foundational information presented throughout the book and offers a forward-looking view of the field. We glance toward the future and provide commentary on what we see to be the upcoming directions and challenges in the field of VHAIs.

Conclusion

Historical trends and current empirical research attest to the long-lasting and complex affinity shared between humans and animals. In this introductory chapter, we positioned HAI as an overarching field under which is situated the subfield of VHAIs. We argued for the relevance of VHAIs in light of the shifting nature of our social and work-related interactions and the current Covid-19 pandemic. We also discussed key theoretical frameworks guiding HAI research, and we set the stage for this book's exploration of the varied pathways and content elucidating people's virtual interactions with animals. We now turn to a review of research examining the benefits for people over the life course of owning a companion animal and/or interacting with animals such as therapy animals. We will then be well-positioned to explore nuances in virtual contexts shared by animals and people and to consider best practices for transferring in-person HAI to a virtual context. We hope that this book will inform and inspire researchers, educators, and practitioners alike to consider how they might facilitate virtual interactions between animals and diverse learners.

References

Adams, C. J. (2015). *The sexual politics of meat: A feminist-vegetarian critical theory*. Bloomsbury Publishing. (Original work published 1990)

Adams, M. (2018). Towards a critical psychology of human-animal relations. *Social and Personality Psychology Compass*, *12*(4), e12375. https://doi.org/10.1111/spc3.12375

American Pet Products Association. (2022). *Pet industry market size, trends & ownership statistics*. Retrieved June 13, 2022, from www.americanpetproducts.org/press_industrytrends.asp

American Veterinary Association. (1998). Statement from the committee on the human-animal bond. *Journal of the American Veterinary Medical Association*, *212*, 1675.

Amiot, C. E., & Bastian, B. (2015). Toward a psychology of human-animal relations. *Psychological Bulletin*, *141*, 6–47. https://doi.org/10.1037/a0038147

Barker, S. B., Barker, R. T., McCain, N. L., & Schubert, C. M. (2016). A randomized cross-over exploratory study of the effect of visiting therapy dogs on college student stress before final exams. *Anthrozoös*, *29*(1), 35–46. https://doi.org/10.1080/08927936.2015.1069988

Beck, A. M. (2014). The biology of the human – animal bond. *Animal Frontiers*, *4*(3), 32–36. https://doi.org/10.2527/af.2014-0019

Beck, A. M., & Katcher, A. H. (1996). *Between pets and people: The importance of animal companionship*. Purdue University Press.

Bekoff, M. (2014). *Rewilding our hearts: Building pathways of compassion and coexistence*. New World Library.

Binfet, J. T., Green, F. L. L., & Draper, Z. A. (2022). The importance of client-canine contact in canine-assisted interventions: A randomized controlled trial. *Anthrozoös*, *35*, 1–22. https://doi.org/10.1080/08927936.2021.1944558

Binfet, J.-T., & Hartwig, E. K. (2020). *Canine-assisted interventions: A comprehensive guide to credentialing therapy dog teams*. Routledge.

Bowlby, J. (1969). *Attachment and loss, Vol. 1. Attachment*. Basic Books.

Cobb, S. (1976). Social support as a moderator of life stress. *Psychosomatic Medicine*, *38*(5), 300–314. https://doi.org/10.1097/00006842-197609000-00003

Cohen, S., & Wills, T. A. (1985). Stress, social support, and the buffering hypothesis. *Psychological Bulletin*, *98*(2), 310–357. https://doi.org/10.1037/0033-2909.98.2.310

Crossman, M. K. (2017). Effects of interactions with animals on human psychological distress. *Journal of Clinical Psychology*, *73*(7), 761–784. https://doi.org/10.1002/jclp.22410

Crossman, M. K., & Kazdin, A. E. (2015). Animal visitation programs in colleges and universities: An efficient model for reducing student stress. In A. H. Fine (Ed.), *Handbook on animal-assisted therapy:*

Foundations and guidelines for animal-assisted interventions (4th ed., pp. 333–337). Elsevier Academic Press. https://doi.org/10.1016/b978-0-12-801292-5.00024-9

Dell, C., Williamson, L., McKenzie, H., Carey, B., Cruz, M., Gibson, M., & Pavelich, A. (2021). A commentary about lessons learned: Transitioning a therapy dog program online during the Covid-19 pandemic. *Animals, 11*, 914. https://doi.org/10.3390/ani11030914

Eddy, J., Hart, L. A., & Boltz, R. P. (2001). The effects of service dogs on social acknowledgments of people in wheelchairs. *The Journal of Psychology, 122*(1), 39–45. https://doi.org/10.1080/00223980.1988.10542941

Fine, A. H. (2014). *Our faithful companions: Exploring the essence of our kinship with animals.* Alpine.

Fine, A. H., & Chastain Griffin, T. (2022). Protecting animal welfare in animal-assisted intervention: Our ethical obligation. *Seminars in Speech and Language, 43*(1). https://doi.org/10.1055/s-0041-1742099

Fine, A. H., & Ferrell, J. (2021). Conceptualizing the human – animal bond and animal-assisted interventions. In J. M. Peralta & A. H. Fine (Eds.), *The welfare of animals in animal-assisted interventions: Foundations and best practice methods* (pp. 21–41). Springer. https://doi.org/10.1007/978-3-030-69587-3_2

Fine, A. H., Tedeshi, P., & Elvove, E. (2015). Forward thinking: The evolving field of human-animal interactions. In A. H. Fine (Ed.), *Handbook on animal-assisted therapy: Foundations and guidelines for animal-assisted interventions* (pp. 21–35). Elsevier Academic Press. https://doi.org/10.1016/B978-0-12-801292-5.00003-1

Fine, A. H., & Weaver, S. J. (2018). The human – animal bond and animal-assisted intervention. In M. van den Bosch & W. Bird (Eds.), *Oxford textbook of nature and public health: The role of nature in improving the health of a population, Oxford Textbooks in Public Health* (pp. 132–138). Oxford. https://doi.org/10.1093/med/9780198725916.003.0028

Gee, N. R., Griffin, J. A., & McCardle, P. (2017). Human – animal interaction research in school settings: Current knowledge and future directions. *AERA Open, 3*(3). https://doi.org/10.1177/2332858417724346

Gee, N. R., Rodriguez, K. E., Fine, A. H., & Trammell, J. P. (2021). Dogs supporting human health and well-being: A biopsychosocial approach. *Frontiers in Veterinary Science, 8.* https://doi.org/10.3389/fvets.2021.630465

Guest, C. M., Collis, G. M., & McNicholas, J. (2006). Hearing dogs: A longitudinal study of social and psychological effects on deaf and hard-of-hearing recipients. *Journal of Deaf Studies and Deaf Education, 11*(2), 252–261. https://doi.org/10.1093/deafed/enj028

Hamza, C. A., Ewing, L., Heath, N. L., & Goldstein, A. L. (2021). When social isolation is nothing new: A longitudinal study on psychological distress during COVID-19 among university students with and without preexisting mental health concerns. *Canadian Psychology/Psychologie Canadienne, 62*(1), 20–30. https://doi.org/10.1037/cap0000255

Handlin, L., Hydbring-Sandberg, E., Nilsson, A., Ejdebäck, M., Jansson, A., & Uvnäs-Moberg, K. (2011). Short-term interaction between dogs and their owners: Effects on oxytocin, cortisol, insulin and heart rate – an exploratory study. *Anthrozoös, 24*(3), 301–315. https://doi.org/10.2752/175303711x13045914865385

Haraway, D. J. (2008). *When species meet.* University of Minnesota Press.

Ho, J., Hussain, S., & Sparagano, O. (2021). Did the COVID-19 pandemic spark a public interest in pet adoption? *Frontiers in Veterinary Science, 8*, 647308. https://doi.org/10.3389/fvets.2021.647308

Howell, T. J., Nieforth, L., Thomas-Pino, C., Samet, L., Agbonika, S., . . . Bennett, P. (2022). Defining terms used for animals working in support roles for people with support needs. *Animals, 12*(15), 1975. https://doi.org/10.3390/ani12151975

Hupcey, J. E. (1998). Social support: Assessing conceptual coherence. *Qualitative Health Research, 8*(3), 304–318. https://doi.org/10.1177/104973239800800302

Insurance Research Council. (2022). www.insurance-research.org

International Association of Human-Animal Interaction Organisations, White Paper on Animal Assisted Interventions. (2018). https://iahaio.org/wp/wp-content/uploads/2017/05/iahaio-white-paper-final-nov-24-2014.pdf (Original work published 2014)

Janssens, M., Janssens, E., Eshuis, J., Lataster, J., Simons, M., Reijnders, J., & Jacobs, N. (2021). Companion animals as buffer against the impact of stress on affect: An experience sampling study. *Animals, 11*(8), 2171. https://doi.org/10.3390/ani11082171

Kahn, P. H., Severson, R. L., & Ruckert, J. H. (2009). The human relation with nature and technological nature. *Current Directions in Psychological Science, 18*(1), 37–42. https://doi.org/10.1111/j.1467-8721.2009.01602.x

Kaparounaki, C. K., Patsali, M. E., Mousa, D.-P. V., Papadopoulou, E. V. K., Papadopoulou, K. K. K., & Fountoulakis, K. N. (2020). University students' mental health amidst the COVID-19 quarantine in Greece. *Psychiatry Research, 290*, 113111. https://doi.org/10.1016/j.psychres.2020.113111

Kellert, S. R., & Wilson, E. O. (1993). *The biophilia hypothesis*. Island Press.

Kruger, K. A., & Serpell, J. A. (2006). Animal-assisted interventions in mental health: Definitions and theoretical foundations. In A. H. Fine (Ed.), *Handbook on animal-assisted therapy: Theoretical foundations and guidelines for practice* (pp. 21–38). Academic Press. https://doi.org/10.1016/b978-0-12-381453-1.10003-0

Louv, R. (2008). *Last child in the woods: Saving our children from nature-deficit disorder*. Algonquin Books of Chapel Hill.

Marino, L. (2012). Construct validity of animal-assisted therapy and activities: How important is the animal in AAT? *Anthrozoös, 25*(Supp. 1). https://doi.org/10.2752/175303712x13353430377219

Matsuoka, A. K., & Sorenson, J. (2018). *Critical animal studies: Towards trans-species social justice*. Rowman & Littlefield International.

McElwain, C. (2020). *Latest Canadian pet population figures released: Press releases*. Latest Canadian Pet Population Figures Released | Press Releases | Canadian Animal Health Institute (CAHI). Retrieved June 13, 2022, from www.cahi-icsa.ca/press-releases/latest-canadian-pet-population-figures-released

Mueller, M. K. (2014). Human-animal interaction as a context for positive youth development: A relational developmental systems approach to constructing human-animal interaction theory and research. *Human Development, 57*(1), 5–25. https://doi.org/10.1159/000356914

Myrick, J. G. (2015). Emotion regulation, procrastination, and watching cat videos online: Who watches internet cats, why, and to what effect? *Computers in Human Behavior, 52*, 168–176. https://doi.org/10.1016/j.chb.2015.06.001

Nagasawa, M., Mitsui, S., En, S., Ohtani, N., Ohta, M., Sakuma, Y., Onaka, T., Mogi, K., & Kikusui, T. (2015). Oxytocin-gaze positive loop and the coevolution of human-dog bonds. *Science, 348*(6232), 333–336. https://doi.org/10.1126/science.1261022

Odendaal, J. S. J., & Meintjes, R. A. (2003). Neurophysiological correlates of affiliative behaviour between humans and dogs. *The Veterinary Journal, 165*(3), 296–301. https://doi.org/10.1016/s1090-0233(02)00237-x

O'Haire, M. (2010). Companion animals and human health: Benefits, challenges, and the road ahead. *Journal of Veterinary Behavior, 5*(5), 226–234. https://doi.org/10.1016/j.jveb.2010.02.002

Parbery-Clark, C., Lubamba, M., Tanner, L., & McColl, E. (2021). Animal-assisted interventions for the improvement of mental health outcomes in higher education students: A systematic review of randomised controlled trials. *International Journal of Environmental Research and Public Health, 18*(20), 10768. https://doi.org/10.3390/ijerph182010768

Payne, E., Bennett, P. C., & McGreevy, P. D. (2015). Current perspectives on attachment and bonding in the dog-human dyad. *Psychology Research and Behavior Management, 8*, 71–79. https://doi.org/10.2147/PRBM.S74972

Pendry, P., & Vandagriff, J. L. (2019). Animal Visitation Program (AVP) reduces cortisol levels of university students: A randomized controlled trial. *AERA Open, 5*(2). https://doi.org/10.1177/2332858419852592

Potts, A. (2010). Introduction: Combating speciesism in psychology and feminism. *Feminism & Psychology, 20*, 291–301. https://doi.org/10.1177%2F0959353510368037

Rault, J.-L. (2015). Pets in the digital age: Live, robot, or virtual? *Frontiers in Veterinary Science, 2*. https://doi.org/10.3389/fvets.2015.00011

Rault, J.-L., van den Munkhof, M., & Buisman-Pijlman, F. T. (2017). Oxytocin as an indicator of psychological and social well-being in domesticated animals: A critical review. *Frontiers in Psychology, 8*. https://doi.org/10.3389/fpsyg.2017.01521

Reeves, B., & Nass, C. (1996). *The media equation: How people treat computers, television, and new media like real people and places*. Center for the Study of Language and Information, Cambridge University Press.

Santaniello, A., Dicé, F., Carratú, R. C., Amato, A., Fioretti, A., & Menna, L. F. (2020). Methodological and terminological issues in animal-assisted interventions: An umbrella review of systematic reviews. *Animals*, *10*, 759. https://doi:10.3390/ani10050759

Schaefer, C., Coyne, J. C., & Lazarus, R. S. (1981). The health-related functions of social support. *Journal of Behavioral Medicine*, *4*(4), 381–406. https://doi.org/10.1007/bf00846149

Schuck, S. E. B., & Fine, A. H. (2017). School-based animal-assisted interventions for children with deficits in executive function. In N. R. Gee, A. H. Fine, & P. McCardle (Eds.), *How animals help students learn: Research and practice for educators and mental health professionals* (pp. 69–82). Routledge/Taylor & Francis Group. https://doi.org/10.4324/9781315620619-6

Serpell, J. (1996). *In the company of animals: A study of human-animal relationships*. Cambridge University Press.

Shapiro, K. (2020). Human-animal studies: Remembering the past, celebrating the present, troubling the future. *Society and Animals*, *28*(7), 797–833. https://doi.org/10.1163/15685306-bja10029

Tang, W., Hu, T., Yang, L., & Xu, J. (2020). The role of alexithymia in the mental health problems of home-quarantined university students during the COVID-19 pandemic in China. *Personality and Individual Differences*, *165*, 110131. https://doi.org/10.1016/j.paid.2020.110131

Thielke, L. E., & Udell, M. A. R. (2020). Characterizing human – dog attachment relationships in foster and shelter environments as a potential mechanism for achieving mutual wellbeing and success. *Animals*, *10*, 67. https://doi.org/10.3390/ani10010067

Wang, C., & Zhao, H. (2020). The impact of COVID-19 on anxiety in Chinese university students. *Frontiers in Psychology*, *11*, 1168. https://doi.org/10.3389/fpsyg.2020.01168

Wilks, S. E., & Spivey, C. A. (2010). Resilience in undergraduate social work students: Social support and adjustment to academic stress. *Social Work Education*, *29*(3), 276–288. https://doi.org/10.1080/02615470902912243

Wilson, E. O. (1984). *Biophilia*. Harvard University Press.

Wohlfarth, R., Mutschler, B., Beetz, A., Kreuser, F., & Korsten-Reck, U. (2013). Dogs motivate obese children for physical activity: Key elements of a motivational theory of animal-assisted interventions. *Frontiers in Psychology*, *4*. https://doi.org/10.3389/fpsyg.2013.00796

World Health Organization. (2021). *Mental health atlas 2020*. Retrieved June 13, 2022, from www.who.int/publications-detail-redirect/9789240036703

Zhou, Z., Yin, D., & Gao, Q. (2020). Sense of presence and subjective well-being in online pet watching: The moderation role of loneliness and perceived stress. *International Journal of Environmental Research and Public Health*, *17*(23), 9093. https://doi.org/10.3390/ijerph17239093

2 From In-Person to Virtual Human-Animal Interactions

An Overview

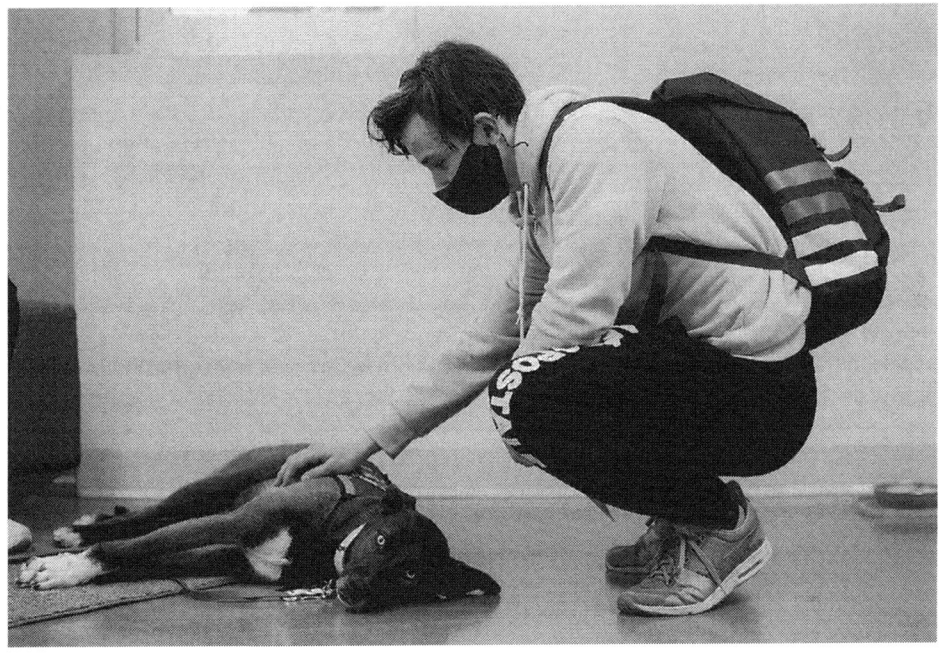

Figure 2.1 A college student spends time with therapy dog Luna

Source: Adam Lauzé – Sarah Lauzé Photography

Scenario

I live my life online, so why do I have to go to an in-person session?

Jacob could hear his Dad's voice telling him, "The last thing you want to do is the first thing you should do." He'd been in his dorm room all week playing online video games with his old high school friends, ordering food to his room, shopping on Amazon, and barely attending classes. He knew his mental health was suffering and that soon his grades would follow. He'd seen emails advertising a stress-reduction therapy dog program on campus and heard students on his floor talking about spending time with therapy dogs to "feel better." Given he missed his family dog back home, Jacob figured he'd

DOI: 10.4324/9781003327868-2

give it a try. Arriving to the program, he sees that he's not the only one who thought this would be a good idea and finds the long line to access the dogs an immediate turnoff. "If I can socialize, order my food, and shop online, why can't I spend time with therapy dogs online?"

Questions for Reflection

1. How might a virtual session with a therapy dog be structured?
2. Are virtual interactions as beneficial as in-person visits?
3. For whom might virtual canine interactions work best?
4. What are the benefits of human-animal interactions?
5. Are virtual HAI sessions an effective way of supporting learners in remote settings?

This scenario depicts a typical situation on college campuses where the demand for access to therapy dogs can often outweigh the capacity of the program to provide it. Jacob's frustration, especially as someone with already compromised well-being, is understandable. What is perhaps most typically appealing about many organized human-animal activities and visitation programs is their casual or informal nature. Certainly, on-campus dog visitation programs are often touted as low-barrier and easy access (Binfet et al., 2022). Many such programs do not require preregistration or a user fee. Taken together, these factors help create optimal conditions for individuals to make use of, or access, these programs as part of efforts to support their mental well-being (see Bailey, 2023 for a recent scoping review of on-campus AAIs). This chapter begins with an overview of in-person HAIs laying the foundation for an overview of VHAIs, something Jacob in our opening scenario would surely have relished.

Human-Animal Interactions 101

What Are Human-Animal Interactions?

Human-Animal Interactions (HAI) describe a wide spectrum of interactions and relationships between animals and humans and are of growing interest to researchers, the general public and the media.

(Ratschen et al., 2020, p. 2)

As noted in our introductory chapter, despite the plethora of published research and applied programs offered, definitions of HAIs can be challenging to find. This definition by Ratschen and colleagues (2020) offers an explanation of HAIs and speaks to the broad range of possibilities of interactions and relationships that might fall under this overarching term. As outlined in Chapter 1, captured under the term HAI are topics of the *human-animal bond* (HAB) and *animal-assisted interventions* (AAIs) among others. Of particular import for this book is the field of AAIs. Parbery-Clark and colleagues (2021) describe AAI as an: "umbrella term that describes the use of various animal species in numerous ways that are beneficial to humans, and includes Animal-Assisted Therapy (AAT), Animal-Assisted Education (AAE), Animal-Assisted Activity (AAA) and more recently, Animal-Assisted Coaching (AAC)" (p. 10768). Though we take exception with these authors' phrasing that refers to animals as being "used," their definition nevertheless illustrates the breadth and scope of HAI iterations captured by this term.

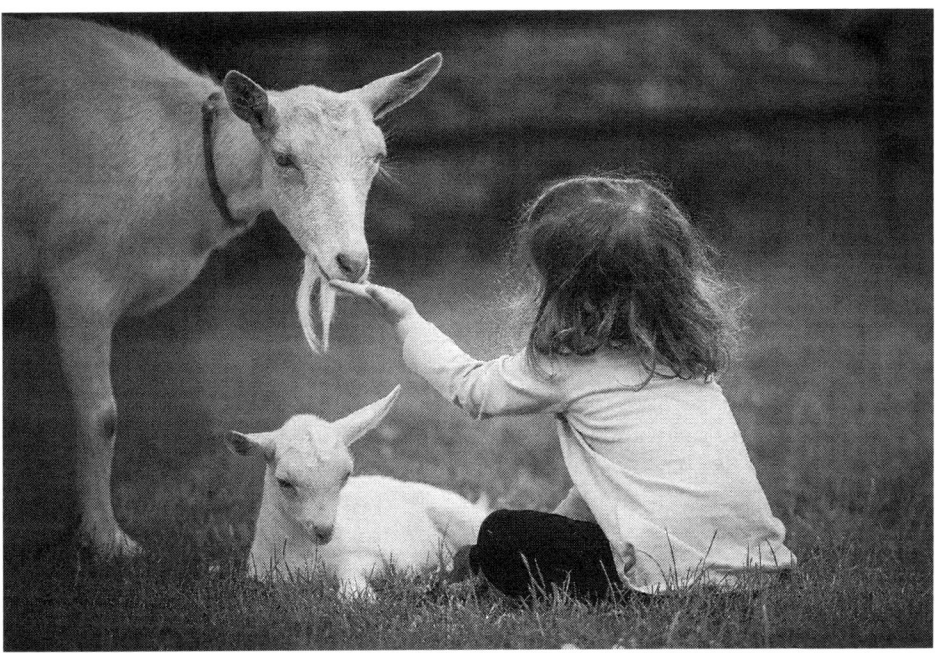

Figure 2.2 A young child introduces herself to a goat and her offspring

Source: Pixabay

Variability in Human-Animal Interactions

A review of publications on the topic of HAIs reveals ample variability in the species we see participating in interventions, the human populations served, the length and duration of interventions themselves, the expertise of researchers or program personnel administering and overseeing interventions, and the use of measures to determine efficacy. Bert and colleagues (2016) differentiate *animal-assisted therapy* (AAT) from *animal-assisted activities* (AAA) and describe the latter as follows: "the differences between AAT and Animal-Assisted Activity (AAA) [is that AAA is (sic)] less structured and mainly composed by pet visitation" (p. 696). These authors offer further elaboration and describe AAAs as: "These kind of activities are in general spontaneous, grouping several patients, and poorly standardized with regard to duration and type of activities" (p. 696). A review of the extant HAI anthrozoological, psychological, and educational literature reveals ample variability that makes refuting Bert and colleagues' description difficult. Certainly, advances have been made, and we're seeing increased transparency in researchers' descriptions of interventions and participants, yet additional detail is needed. What follows next is an overview of the variability in HAIs, followed by a call to increase transparency in the descriptions of HAIs implemented across settings.

Species Variability

As noted in Chapter 1, a review of seminal and recent publications exploring and examining HAIs reveals a propensity for animal participants to be canines or equines as these species are known to have dispositions that make them easy to work with: They respond more or less predictably to the direction of handlers, they may work in close proximity to other dogs/horses, they may adapt to varied settings and clientele, and they have broad appeal, readily drawing in clients. Dogs, in particular, are frequently employed within AAIs, and much has been written on the characteristics of therapy dogs, for instance, that helps determine their suitability for AAI-related work (for a review, see Hartwig & Binfet, 2019). Given our familiarity and experience working with therapy dogs, throughout our book we lean heavily on dog-centric AAI research to support our VHAI insights and arguments, recognizing that dogs are but one species with whom researchers and practitioners collaborate in delivering HAIs. It warrants mention that accessing well-trained therapy dog-handler teams often poses a challenge and, as one example, in the B.A.R.K. office at the University of British Columbia, the requests for therapy dogs to participate in community-based programming, especially in local schools, surpasses our ability to provide dog-handler teams.

Still prevalent, yet less evident, in the AAI literature are horses, and a variety of therapeutic interaction and/or riding programs have been developed, implemented, and evaluated across varied contexts (e.g., prison settings, residential care facilities for seniors). In recent innovative research titled "The potential for equine-assisted psychotherapy for treating trauma in Australian Aboriginal peoples," researchers Bennet and Woodman (2019) collaborate with therapy horses to address issues of disparity, diversity, and decolonization in their crafting of a culturally responsive therapeutic AAI. These researchers define equine-assisted psychotherapy as "an experiential therapy that facilitates interactions between horses and humans, in sessions designed to obtain therapy goals" (Bennet & Woodman, 2019, p. 1046). Though an example of a *psychotherapeutic* intervention that extends beyond informal AAIs and requires advanced training on the part of the therapist, much can be gleaned from this work to inform the design and delivery of HAIs. Bennet and Woodman argue that individuals delivering AAIs for Aboriginal clients (or within Aboriginal cultural contexts) must first "understand their own cultural identity and background, including values, assumptions, and expectations" (p. 1052). Thus, both reflection and introspection are required prior to AAI participation – not only a recommendation for working with Aboriginal clients but as a way of ensuring all clients' backgrounds and cultures are considered and respected in the design and delivery of the HAI.

Recommendations for tailoring AAIs to Aboriginal contexts include being aware of the diversity within Aboriginal cultures, the value of Aboriginal knowledge and skills, traditional protocols, and "Aboriginal Country and Aboriginal levels of government" (Bennet & Woodman, 2019, p. 1052). Bennet and Woodman argue that the introduction of AAIs for Aboriginal peoples is in strong alignment with the core values/principles of Aboriginal culture where animals (and nature more broadly) are pivotally situated. Extending our lens further to the principles guiding Indigenous research, the work of Pidgeon and Riley (2021) informs our thinking around how to conduct AAI research that honors Indigenous people and culture. These researchers argue that Indigenous research should uphold the following principles:

> Indigenous research practices are based on *respect* for Indigenous ways of knowing and being (Nakata, 2003), relevance to the community/Nation, *reciprocity* in research processes, and *responsibility* in the relationships between researchers and the community (Pidgeon, 2018; Pidgeon & Hardy Cox, 2002).
>
> (Pidgeon & Riley, 2021, p. 3)

Thus, AAI research within this context would honor prior knowledge and understanding of animals, the role of animals within Indigenous culture, and the relation between animals and Indigenous people. Also, AAI research within this context would be characterized by an intervention of importance to the community in which it is being conducted (versus uniquely important for the researcher),

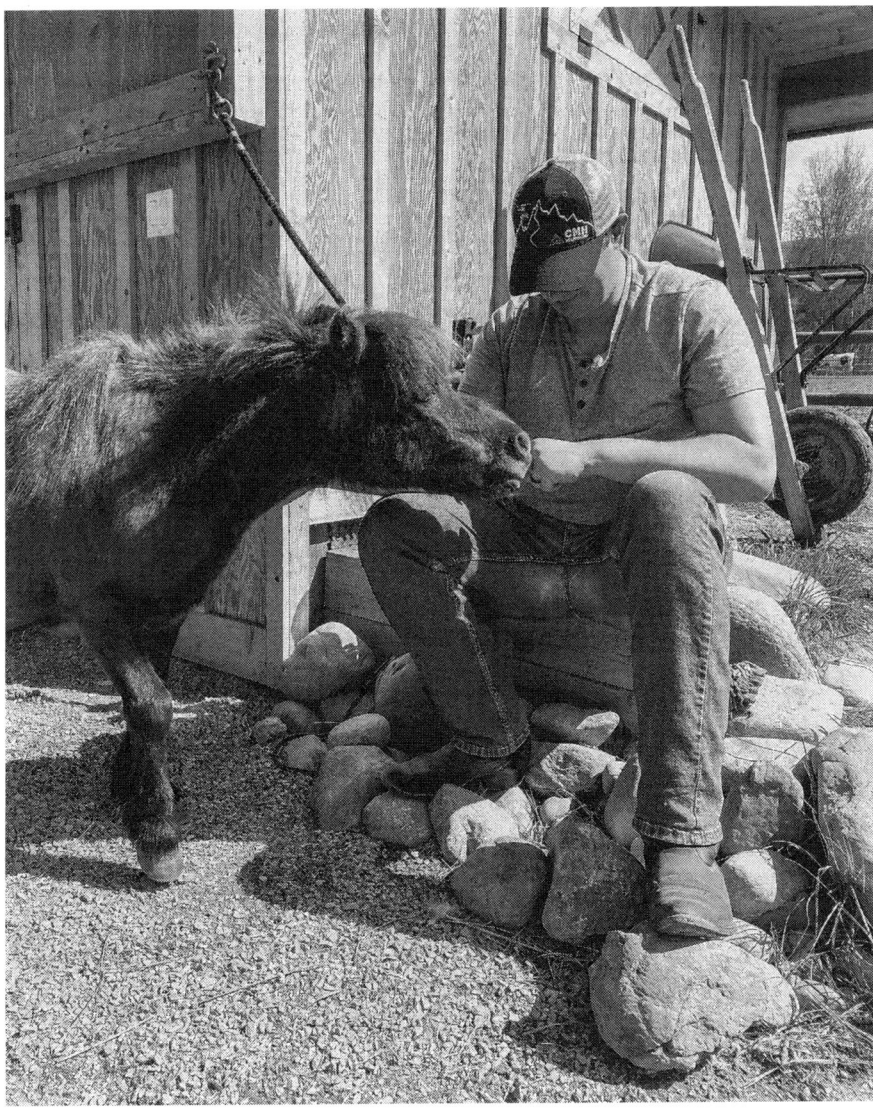

Figure 2.3 In which hand is the treat? A horse-human interaction

Source: F. L. L. Green Photography

with findings that are shared openly and broadly within the community, and a researcher who is committed to building or nurturing relationships throughout and beyond data collection.

Showcasing other equine-assisted interventions (EAI) is the work of Kinney and colleagues (2019), whose recent systematic mapping review illustrates the breadth of equine-themed research in support of veterans spanning 1980 to 2017. In concert with our earlier reporting around the variability in interventions, these authors recommend future research consider "the theoretical development of equine-assisted interventions for veterans and thoroughly describe the participants, components of the intervention, factors contributing to attrition, and optimal dose-response relationships" (Kinney et al., 2019, p. 1).

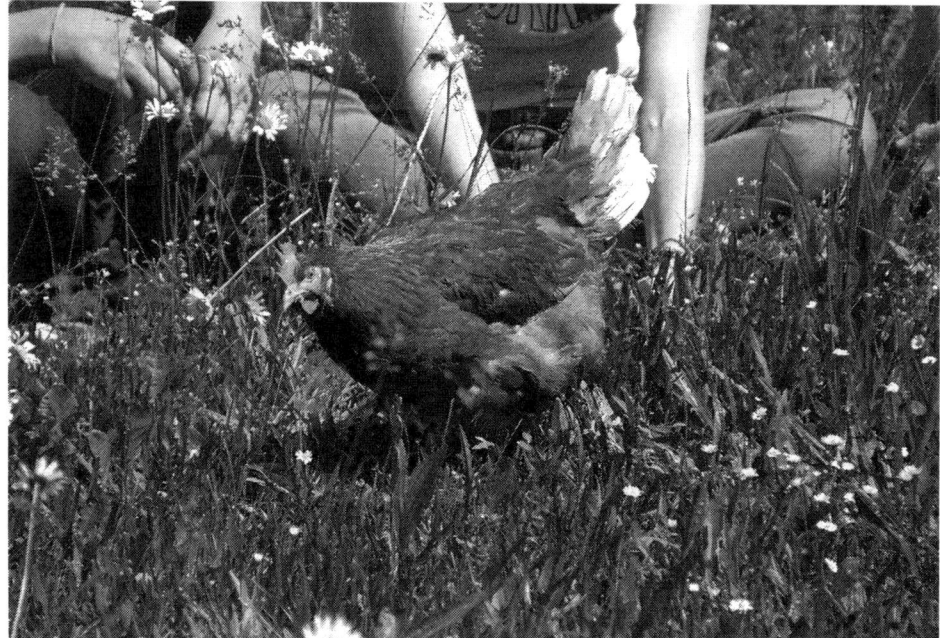

Figure 2.4 Interacting with a hen

Source: Pixabay

Though dogs and horses dominate the AAI landscape, other species have participated in AAIs or programs. The University of Michigan's BioKIDS program sees children learn about African snails (BioKIDS, n.d.) and other researchers have collaborated with guinea pigs (O'Haire et al., 2013), goats (Harada et al., 2019), and chickens (Hodgson et al., 2022). To this latter species, spearheaded by Hodgson and colleagues (2013) at Northumbria University, a program titled "HENPOWER" was conceptualized to support seniors in a residential care facility. The aim of this program was to "enhance social interaction, enjoyment of life, wellbeing, and quality of life" (p. 7) by providing opportunities for residents to interact with hens.

Variability in Populations Served

A review of published AAI research reveals that this is a modality that is adaptable to, and accessible by, a wide variety of human clients. In the referenced systematic review by Bert and colleagues (2016), a review of 432 AAI publications revealed that AAIs within hospital contexts serve primarily children, psychiatric populations, and elderly patients. Casting an eye more broadly and to varied contexts, we see programs implemented for but not limited to the following populations (see Table 2.1).

Variability in Intervention Dose and Duration

Although there is variability in both the species collaborating in interventions and the clients supported by interventions, there is perhaps the greatest variability found in both the duration of the intervention comprising a session (i.e., the number of minutes that animals interact with human clients) and the duration or number of sessions offered over time that

Table 2.1 Examples Showcasing the Variability in Human Clients and Animal Species Participating in Human-Animal Interventions

Population Served	Species	Citation
Children	African Snails	BioKIDS (n.d.)
	Companion Animals	Tardif-Williams & Bosacki, 2015
	Dogs	Harris & Binfet, 2022
		Rousseau & Tardif-Williams, 2019
	Guinea Pigs	O'Haire et al., 2013
	Horses	Mukherjee, 2020
	Rabbits	Molnár et al., 2020
Children with Special Needs	Dogs	Esteves & Stokes, 2008
		Lobato Rincón et al., 2021
Children & Adults	Goats	Toshihide et al., 2019
Adolescents	Dogs	Mueller et al., 2021
College Students	Dogs	Barker et al., 2016; Binfet et al.,
	Dogs & Cats	2018; Pendry et al., 2018; Pendry & Vandagriff, 2019
Adults	Horses	Bennet & Woodman, 2019; Kinney et al., 2019
Senior Citizens	Llamas	Kingson, 2019
Adults with Special Needs	Dogs	Wijker et al., 2020
Law Enforcement Officers	Dogs	Binfet et al., 2020
Psychiatric Patients	Dogs	Scheck et al., 2022
Inmates	Dogs	Cooke & Farrington, 2016; Villafaina-Dominguez et al., 2020; Deaton, 2005
	Dogs & Horses	
Military Veterans	Horses	Boss et al., 2019

comprise an intervention (i.e., the number of sessions per week, the number of weeks of program delivery). A summary of dose variation used in randomized controlled trials assessing the effects of spending time with therapy dogs published in 2017 illustrates this variability (see Table 2.2 here).

With respect to AAIs collaborating with therapy dogs, we see researchers make use of single sessions, sometimes even abbreviated single sessions (see Barker et al., 2016; Binfet et al., 2022, and Crossman et al., 2015 here for illustrations) and others offer more comprehensive AAI programming that sees the delivery of multiple sessions spanning several weeks. In an innovative study out of the B.A.R.K. lab at the University of British Columbia, instead of prescribing participants a predetermined dosage/duration, we allowed participants to determine the length of the interaction with therapy dogs they felt was needed in order for them to reduce their stress. Analyzing the length of time 1,960 undergraduate students spent with therapy dogs revealed visits of 35 minutes with women staying, on average 2 minutes longer than their male counterparts (see Binfet et al., 2018).

Readers curious to learn of the benefits to well-being arising from AAIs are reminded to be critical consumers of AAI research (for a recent discussion of rigour in AAI research, see Huber et al., 2022 for their systematic review and meta-analysis). There are few standards of practice in place with regard to the design and delivery of AAIs to elicit well-being benefits. Thus, despite sweeping claims that AAIs are effective in eliciting a whole host of well-being outcomes, the critical consumer of AAI research will be quick to ascertain the intervention duration as an indicator of methodological and empirical rigour. Relatedly, we must use caution in

Table 2.2 Variations in Dose Intervention in Randomized Controlled Trials Employing Canine-Assisted Therapy

Study	Dose Intervention (min)	Number of Sessions per Week	Duration of Intervention (weeks)	Number of Participants
Barker et al. (2015)	10	1	1	40
Barker et al. (2016)	15	1	1	57
Binfet & Passmore (2016)	45	1	8	44
Chu et al. (2009)	50	1	8	30
Crossman & Kazdin (2015)	7 to 10	1	1	67
Fung & Leung (2014)	20	3	7	10
Grajfoner et al. (2016)	20	1	1	132
Havener et al. (2001)	—	1	1	40
Johnson et al. (2008)	15	3	4	30
Martin & Farnum (2002)	15	3	15	10
Schuck et al. (2015)	120 to 150	2	12	24
Vagnoli et al. (2015)	—	1	1	50
Villalta-Gil et al. (2009)	45	2	25	21

Note: — indicates data not reported.

Source: reprinted with permission from *Anthrozoös*

comparing studies or aggregating findings from across studies given the variability in methodological approaches, especially regarding the duration of the intervention itself.

Variability in the Training of Program Personnel

Just as there is variability in the duration of session, so, too, do we see ample variability in the screening and training of animal-handler teams. This is an especially important dimension of AAIs as the quality of training received by teams along with their experience can impact the quality of the AAIs they facilitate. A well-trained handler, for example, who is able to ask open-ended prompts to clients followed by active empathic listening, can enhance the experience of clients participating in an AAI. Increasingly, researchers are reporting information regarding handler training and experience with some studies reporting that handlers follow scripts or draw questions from a bank of questions in intervention studies – as a way of levelling the playing field across dog-handler teams when multiple teams participate in an intervention. At the very least, when reporting empirical findings, demographic information regarding the dog-handler teams should be reported (e.g., mean age, mean years volunteer experience in AAIs).

Variability in Methodologies and Measures Used

Obviously, when determining the effects of AAIs on a variety of well-being outcomes, we see researchers frequently employ randomized controlled trials, a rigorous research design that randomly assigns participants to treatment (i.e., time interacting with an animal) or control (i.e., interactions without an animal) conditions and increases the researcher's ability to claim whether the AAI was, in fact, effective. Readers curious to delve further into the topic of variability in HAI research are encouraged to read the recent work of Rodriguez et al. (2021; 2023) that explores the complexities of researching the effects of animal companionship and HAIs.

Certainly, the published AAI research skews to that employing quantitative methodologies; however, there have been calls for additional qualitative research to capture a broader and more comprehensive sense of the client's experience as part of an AAI. Researchers have claimed that qualitative research methods remain underutilized within the field of HAI research and using exploratory qualitative methods stands to enrich the research landscape around understanding all and varied aspects of HAIs (Fournier, 2019; Kazdin, 2017). This argument is raised by Kazdin (2017) in his call for additional qualitative HAI research:

> Qualitative research would readily allow in-depth evaluation of the experiences of clients across different forms of AAI and to see the extent to which commonalities emerge in how the intervention is experienced.
>
> (p. 156)

It merits noting that these research calls also align with interdisciplinary theoretical frameworks such as posthumanism (Haraway, 2008) and critical animal studies (Matsuoka & Sorenson, 2018), as discussed in Chapter 1, that offer new and inspiring ways of thinking about animals and animal-human relationships and that seek to challenge traditional boundaries between humans and animals (Haraway, 2008; Shapiro, 2020).

The Benefits of In-Person Human-Animal Interactions

Though not universally reported across studies, peer-reviewed findings generally attest to both intra- and interpersonal benefits arising from AAIs (see Bert et al., 2016; Huber et al., 2022; and Wagner et al., 2022 for systematic reviews of factors impacting AAI outcomes). This next section provides an overview of some of the key benefits identified for participants' learning, social connectedness, and well-being that arise from interventions that provide opportunities for humans to interact with animals.

Animals Assisting With Learning – Animal-Assisted Education

Just as the broader field of AAIs is flourishing, so, too, is the subsidiary field of animal-assisted education (AAE) that predominantly sees animals working with children in formal and informal educational settings and programs. Often implemented with children with exceptional needs, educators partner with animals to support children in learning, practicing, and mastering a variety of academic and social and emotional goals (for reviews of AAEs, see Hall et al., 2016; Reilly et al., 2020; Sandt, 2020). Not surprisingly and in alignment with the bulk of research conducted in AAIs, therapy dogs are the prevalent species we see partnering in AAEs, and as a testament to their adaptable and flexible nature, we see dogs working in complex and busy school settings to meet the needs of diverse learners.

Certainly, a popular form of AAE is when therapy dogs participate in children's reading activities with the aim of helping children practice reading aloud in a nonthreatening and encouraging environment. Often referred to as *Reading to Dogs* or RTD (Steel, 2023), we see such programs in library settings (e.g., Rousseau & Tardif-Williams, 2019) or classrooms (e.g., Kirnan et al., 2016). Steel (2023) describes the mechanisms at play within RTD as: "Advocates

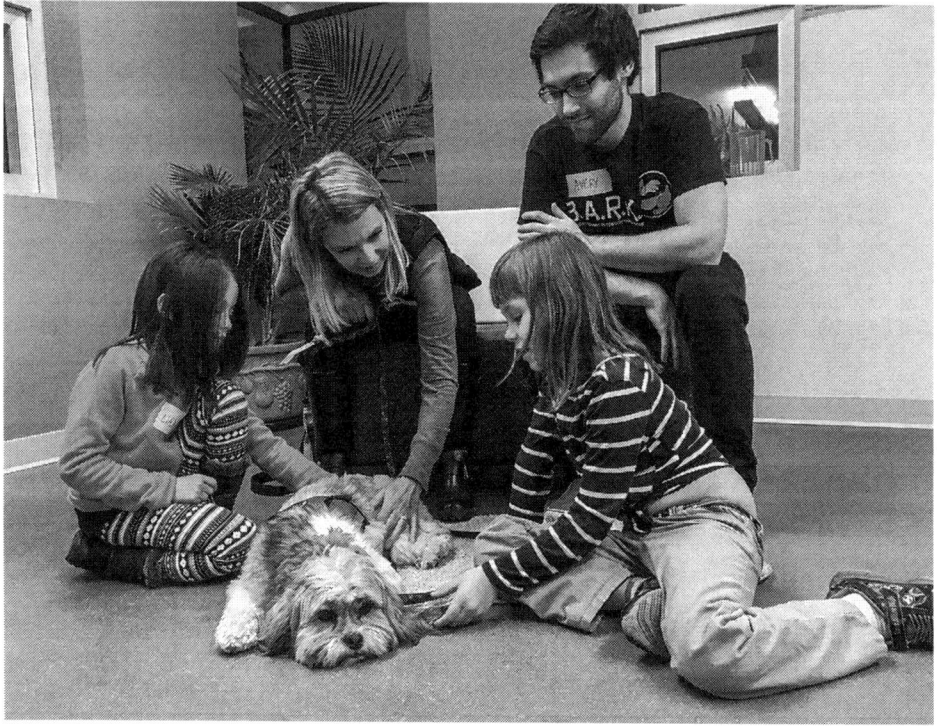

Figure 2.5 Children practicing their social awareness skills alongside therapy dog Murphy in UBC's program *Building Confidence through K9s*

Source: F. L. L. Green Photography

suggest that non-critical listening and unconditional positive regard bestowed on the child by the dog reduce anxiety and improve confidence and attitudes toward reading" (p. 1). The findings attesting to the utility of RTDs in fostering positive reading-related outcomes show promise; however, researchers have made calls for additional rigour to help strengthen causal claims reflecting the efficacy of RTDs (Brelsford et al., 2017; Rodriguez et al., 2023). As is the case with AAIs more broadly, there is variability in how RTDs are implemented with some programs following a predetermined curriculum and others operating informally.

In recent innovative research by Steel (2023), a RTD was adapted for online delivery with 106 school children assigned to reading conditions with or without a dog. Although measures of reading affect, frequency, and well-being were administered pre- and post-participation, no significant differences arising from the virtual RTD program were found. The program was, however, found to be "feasible and practical" when implemented in a virtual format within the context of primary school classrooms (Steel, 2023, p. 9) – that is, the in-person approach could be reimagined for virtual delivery. In contrast to the quantitative findings, qualitative responses from both children and their teachers suggested the virtual RTD program played a role in bolstering children's confidence and reducing nervousness. The author posits that the RTD program boosted students' motivation to read and reading frequency – factors not captured within the confines of the study as they may appear latently. As the adaptation of AAIs to virtual contexts is a complicated undertaking, additional research of this nature assessing the efficacy of in-person programs adapted for a virtual context is needed.

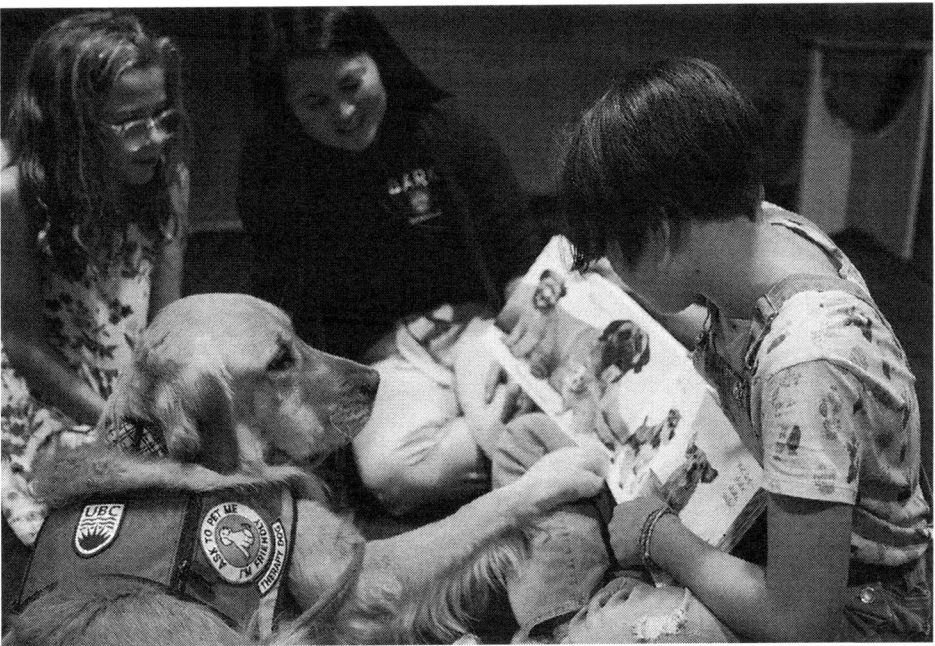

Figure 2.6 Children practice reading to therapy dog Abby

Source: Adam Lauzé – Sarah Lauzé Photography

Animals Assisting With Establishing Connections to Others – Animals as Social Catalysts

Interpersonally, we see animals act as social catalysts (sometimes referred to as social lubricants), connecting people to one another with participants reporting an increase in their perception of their connectedness to others (McNicholas & Collis, 2000; Colarelli et al., 2017). Research findings across studies attest to animals being effective in facilitating interactions across varied contexts and supporting varied clients. One illustration of this is found in the recent research of Barak et al. (2001) who assigned 20 hospitalized elderly patients with chronic schizophrenia to weekly animal interaction sessions with a dog or cat or to a control condition that saw participants engage in reading and discussing current news events. The findings revealed that participants in the animal-interaction condition demonstrated significant pre-to-post-test gains on measures of social-interpersonal interactions and life skills. In their description of their methodology, these researchers describe one role that animals played in fostering communication and socialization: "Patients were encouraged to share feelings of isolation and loneliness by first confiding in their animal companions and later with their group co-members" (Barak et al., 2001, p. 441). We see the animals in this study positioned as therapeutic partners who, in a nonthreatening manner, are able to encourage the sharing of experiences from human-to-animal and extending that to subsequently encourage sharing from human-to-human.

In a recent systematic review by Baird and colleagues (2022), 23 studies exploring the impact of therapy dogs on students' social and emotional well-being were examined. Like many other areas of HAI research, there were discrepant findings attesting to the role therapy dogs played in enhancing varied aspects of students' social and emotional competencies.

However, findings from across studies situated within primary, secondary, and special education contexts, revealed that therapy dogs were perceived by students and educators as improving students' social and communication skills. Additionally, therapy dogs were determined to play a role in both fostering student-to-student connections and student-teacher rapport. "Students also perceived being more confident and positive about themselves as learners and having more positive social interactions and relationships with their teachers (a mutual perception of teachers)" (Baird et al., 2022, p. 198). In addition to intra- and interpersonal gains in social and emotional competencies, therapy dogs working in varied educational settings contributed to improved school climate. This holds implications for student motivation and subsequent learning. Thus, findings from this study suggest that therapy dogs may impact students' own development and growth, their connections and interactions with peers and teachers, and the larger context in which they learn. Readers are directed to a recent scoping review by Chan et al. (2022) that proves a comprehensive overview of AAI and children's social and emotional learning.

Findings such as this are in concert with the biophilia hypothesis (Wilson, 1984), which was introduced in our introductory chapter. Recall that this theory posits that humans are drawn to life and lifelike organisms and that animals, in a calm, resting state, convey a sense of safety or security to people. This, in turn, renders individuals at ease, feeling calm or settled in their environment, and perhaps contributes to them being more open to interacting with others. Building on this sense of safety and security that therapy dogs, in particular, are able to provide, an innovative AAI was conceptualized by Harris and Binfet (2022) that saw children from an urban after-school program participate in a program titled "Building Confidence through K9s." Assigned a dog-handler team and an undergraduate student mentor upon their arrival to the university, 22 children participated in weekly hour-long sessions to learn and practice a series of social and emotional competencies. Purposefully organized as a group intervention, children were paired with other children to comprise their group and, over the course of six weeks, engaged in lessons designed to foster their social confidence. This intervention included practicing introductions both within their group and beyond their group during short excursions out on campus (see Figure 2.6). Similar to the methodology used in the Barak et al. (2001) study described earlier that saw elderly patients first share information with their assigned animal as part of the intervention, here we saw children first practice their social and emotional skills with their assigned therapy dog. The rationale here was that the nonjudgmental and nonthreatening nature of the therapy dogs would encourage children, who may otherwise be reluctant, to engage with their therapy dog and practice their assigned skills. Observations of participants by research assistants and handlers combined with findings from semi-structured interviews with the children themselves revealed the program to be effective in bolstering students' sense of self, their perspective-taking abilities, and their social confidence.

It's not only therapy dogs who have demonstrated a propensity for fostering social connections among people. Horses, too, have been shown to increase humans' social functioning. In a study by Bass et al. (2009), a 12-week horseback riding intervention that saw children with autism (aged 5–10) assigned to either riding a therapy horse ($n = 19$) or assigned to a wait-list control condition ($n = 15$) reported children in the horse condition demonstrated significant improvements in their social motivation (defined as "the extent to which a respondent is generally motivated to engage in social-interpersonal behavior" (Bass et al., 2009, p. 1263). The authors posit that the horses required participants to refocus their attention – to listen to directions and to talk to their horse. Again, we see the animal positioned here as a therapeutic partner, a key agent in the AAI, able to provide a safe foundation upon which participants can both learn about themselves and others.

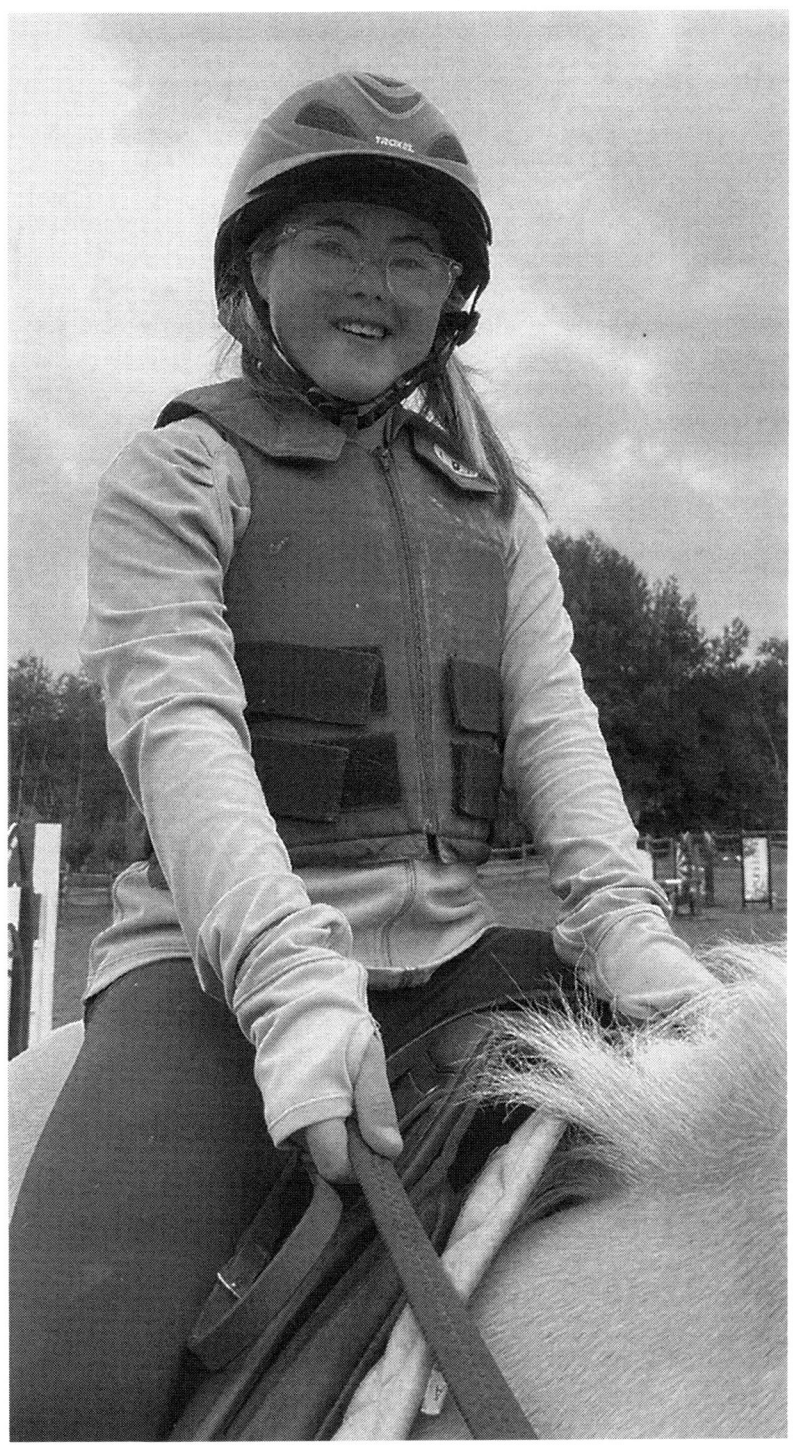

Figure 2.7 A child smiles in delight as she rides a horse

Source: F. L. L. Green Photography

Animal-Assisted Interventions Fostering Well-Being

There is ample variability in how well-being is conceptualized, but generally, we might consider it as a state of being comprised of both positive (e.g., happiness) and negative (e.g., loneliness) dimensions. As researchers working within a broad mental health framework, we lean on the World Health Organization's (2023) Health and Wellbeing subsection definition that describes mental health as "a state of wellbeing in which every individual realizes his or her own potential, can cope with the normal stresses of life, can work productively and fruitfully and is able to make a contribution to his or her community." Arguments have been made to ensure that well-being is conceptualized for specific groups (i.e., children, college students, elderly; Dodd et al., 2021) and certainly, that measures used to assess well-being are normed on samples comparable to the study population in question. These considerations are especially important within the context of AAI research.

Across varied AAIs that feature horses (Boss et al., 2019), cats (Pendry & Vandagriff, 2019), dogs (Binfet et al., 2018; Meints et al., 2022), and other animals (Casey et al., 2017), AAIs have been shown to elicit a host of positive well-being outcomes. We see participants report reductions in their perceptions of both negative dimensions of well-being – including stress (Barker et al., 2016), homesickness (Binfet & Passmore, 2016), anxiety (Crossman et al., 2015; Foerder & Royer, 2021), and negative affect (Binfet et al., 2022) – and positive dimensions of well-being – including self-esteem, happiness, and positive affect (Barker et al., 2016; Binfet et al., 2022; Muckle & Lasikiewicz, 2017). Stress reduction features predominantly in AAI research and increasingly we're seeing researchers measure biomarker indicators of stress such as cortisol (Meints et al., 2022; Pendry & Vandagriff, 2019). A recent systematic review and meta-analysis of 35 AAI studies within higher education contexts by Huber et al. (2022) revealed that AAIs, across studies, are shown to consistently reduce students' anxiety and stress with less consistent evidence found for AAIs impacting students' cognitive and physiological health outcomes.

What's Needed in the Field of Human-Animal Interactions?

Thus far we've established that there is both ample variability in the design and delivery of AAIs and that variability in the claims attesting to the benefits of AAIs (and more broadly HAIs) is evident. We argue in this book that by virtue of the format of virtual AAIs, this variability may be reduced. Next, we discuss virtual programs or interventions featuring HAIs, and we review some of the published research to date examining the delivery and effects of spending time virtually with animals.

From In-Person to Virtual Human-Animal Interactions

The variability found across AAIs discussed at the outset of this chapter may be reduced through offering virtual opportunities to spend time with animals. Virtual AAIs are defined as digital opportunities for passive (i.e., asynchronous) or active (i.e., synchronous) interactions with animals with the purpose of supporting learning, social connections, and well-being. However, despite the variability found across AAIs, they are often restricted by both structure and format (i.e., that interactions are of a predetermined length), as well as delivery. That said, there remains ample variation in what might constitute a virtual human-animal interaction (VHAI), and in our next chapter, we'll examine more closely examples of virtual human-animal connections.

Admittedly, the subfield of VHAI is new and emerging, and, as such, little has been published explicating this approach or elucidating the efficacy of providing virtual opportunities to connect with animals. As we discussed in Chapter 1, Fine et al. (2015) in a chapter titled "Forward thinking: The evolving field of human-animal interactions" positions the (over) use of technology as contributing to "nature deprivation" (p. 28). This latter argument is that humans' propensity to live their lives within digital contexts reduces their opportunities (or interest or desire) to interact with nature. In contrast to Fine et al.'s view positioning technology as detracting from nature, one aim of our book is to illustrate just how technology may be leveraged to provide virtual connections with animals (and, more broadly, nature). Thus, we position technology as a vehicle through which HAIs may be fostered or facilitated – a sort of portal through which HAIs may be offered and made accessible.

But Isn't Touch Essential?

> Previous research has mainly focused on investigating *if* AAIs work but almost entirely ignored the question of *how* it works.
>
> (Wagner et al., 2022, p. 2)

A recent theme in AAI research has been to assess the effect of touch within AAI sessions on well-being outcomes in humans. It is posited that touch between humans and animals optimally bolsters or fosters well-being in humans, contributing to a host of positive outcomes. Next, we review this emerging area of research and then juxtapose the importance of touch vis-à-vis VHAIs.

Despite the burgeoning research examining the effects of spending time with therapy dogs, researchers have yet to identify the mechanisms within interactions that are especially effective

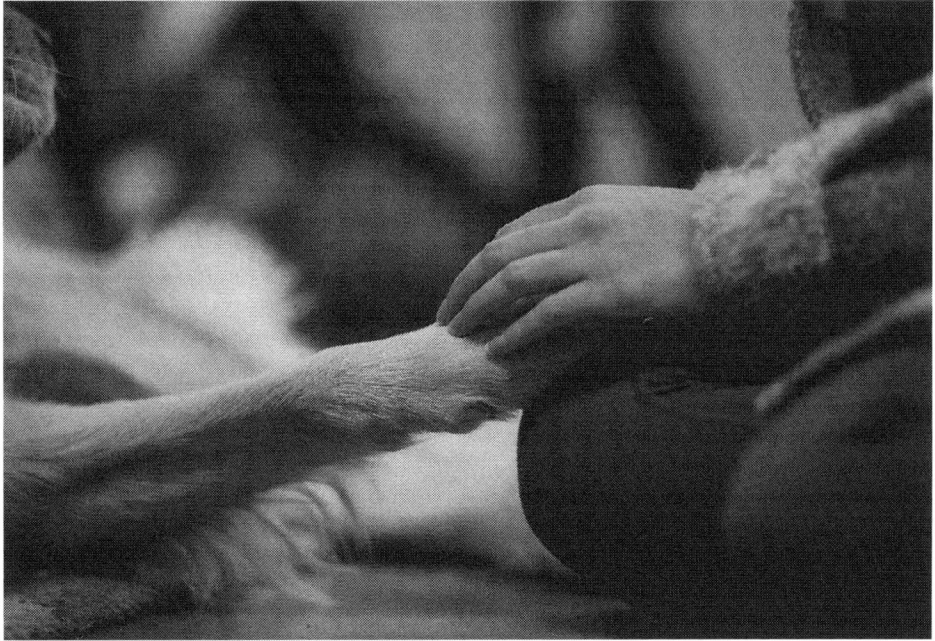

Figure 2.8 The role of touch in animal-assisted interventions

Source: Adam Lauzé – Sarah Lauzé Photography

in eliciting well-being outcomes in participants (Binfet et al., 2022; Wagner et al., 2022). Researchers have more recently begun trying to answer the question – what, within a session, contributes to positive well-being outcomes? Suspecting that touch between the human visitor and the animal is a key and possibly essential element of the HAI, researchers have examined the role of touch as a mechanism within sessions to determine the role it plays in fostering well-being in clients. An early study of 31 boys (aged 7–12) by Beetz et al. (2011) found that children who physically touched a therapy dog as part of their interaction (versus a non-dog/human-only condition and a toy dog condition) had lower salivary cortisol levels. The use of biomarker indicators of well-being is found in a subsequent study by Pendry and Vandagriff (2019) who assessed the effect of a canine-visitation program on college ($N = 249$) students' stress. Students who participated in hands-on petting of dogs (versus students who either observed others petting dogs and cats, viewed images of dogs and cats, or were in a wait-list control condition) experienced significant reductions in their pre-to-post salivary cortisol levels. The role of touch as a variable reducing anxiety was explored in a recent study by Mueller and colleagues (2021) who randomly assigned adolescents ($N = 66$) to a no-touch condition with a dog present, a touch condition with a therapy dog, and a control condition with a toy dog. As summarized by the authors, "We found no evidence that the presence of a real dog, with our without the opportunity to touch it, reduced anxiety of autonomic reactivity or improved cognitive performance relative to the presence of a stuffed dog in the control condition, regardless of levels of preexisting social anxiety" (Mueller et al., 2021, p. 1).

In an effort to explore the role of touch in reducing stress in college students, Binfet and colleagues (2022) conducted a randomized controlled trial of 284 undergraduate students assigned to either a direct hands-on condition that saw them pet a therapy dog for 20 minutes, or a corresponding no-touch condition, or a no-dog condition. Measures of flourishing, positive and negative affect, social connectedness, happiness, campus integration, stress, homesickness, and loneliness were administered pre- and post-interaction. Only participants in the direct touch condition (i.e., those who interacted through constant petting of the therapy dog for 20 minutes) reported significant improvements on all measures of well-being.

Implications of Touch for Virtual Human-Animal Interactions

Although there are exceptions (e.g., Mueller et al., 2021), the findings from studies conducted to date collectively suggest that touch may play a key role in optimizing well-being for visitors to AAI sessions. Recognizing that touch between human visitors and therapy animals is not always possible, for a variety of reasons (e.g., allergies, access to programs), exploring options to facilitate interactions via different modalities helps broaden access to AAIs. In our next chapter, we delve more deeply into the offering of virtual human-animal interactions as one possible alternative to meeting the needs of clients where in-person interactions are impossible or unavailable.

Conclusion

Our aim in this chapter was to provide an overview of AAIs. We first sought to illustrate the variability that exists around the nature and design of interventions, the animals that participate in interventions, and the variability in the outcome variables sought; and second, illustrate how in-person AAIs lay the foundation for creating opportunities for virtual human-animal connections. What follows next is a review of the nascent published research on virtual human-animal interactions at the time of our writing this book.

References

Bailey, K. (2023). A scoping review of campus-based animal-assisted interaction programs for college student mental health. *People and Animals: The International Journal of Research and Practice, 6*(1). https://docs.lib.purdue.edu/paij/vol6/iss1/1

Baird, R., Grové, C., & Berger, E. (2022). The impact of therapy dog son the social and emotional wellbeing of students: A systematic review. *Educational and Developmental Psychologist, 39*(2), 180–208. https://doi.org/10.1080/20590776.2022.2049444

Barak, Y., Savorai, O., Mavashev, S., & Avshalom Beni, A. M. (2001). Animal-assisted therapy for elderly schizophrenic patients: A one-year controlled trial. *The American Journal of Geriatric Psychiatry, 9*(4), 439–442. https://doi.org/10.1097/00019442-200111000-00013

Barker, S. B., Barker, R. T., McCain, N. L., & Schubert, C. M. (2016). A randomized cross-over exploratory study of the effect of visiting therapy dogs on college student stress before final exams. *Anthrozoös, 29*(1), 35–46. https://doi.org/10.1080/08927936.2015.1069988

Bass, M. M., Duchowny, C. A., & Llabre, M. M. (2009). The effect of horseback riding on social functioning in children with autism. *Journal of Autism Development Disorder, 39*(9), 1261–1267. https://doi.org/10.1007/s10803-009-0734-3

Beetz, A., Kotrschal, K., Turner, D. C., Hediger, K., Uvnäs-Moberg, K., & Julius, H. (2011). The effect of a real dog, toy dog and friendly person on insecurely attached children during a stressful task: An exploratory study. *Anthrozoös, 24*(4), 349–368. https://doi.org/10.2752/175303711X13159027359746

Bennet, B., & Woodman, E. (2019). The potential of equine-assisted psychotherapy for treating trauma in Australian Aboriginal peoples. *British Journal of Social Work, 49*, 1049–1058. https://doi.org/10.1093/bjsw/bcz053

Bert, F., Gualano, M. R., Camussi, E., Pieve, G., Voglino, G., & Siliquini, R. (2016). Animal assisted intervention: A systematic review of benefits and risks. *European Journal of Integrative Medicine, 8*, 695–706. https://dx.doi.org/10.1016/j.eujim.2016.05.005

Binfet, J. T., Draper, Z. A., & Green, F. L. L. (2020). Stress reduction in law enforcement officers and staff through a canine-assisted intervention. *Human Animal Interaction Bulletin, 8*(2), 34–52.

Binfet, J. T., Green, F. L. L., & Draper, Z. A. (2022). The importance of client-canine contact in canine-assisted interventions: A randomized controlled trial. *Anthrozoös, 35*, 1–22. https://doi.org/10.1080/08927936.2021.1944558

Binfet, J. T., & Passmore, H. A. (2016). Hounds and homesickness: The effects of an animal-assisted therapeutic intervention for first-year university students. *Anthrozoös, 29*(3), 441–454. https://doi.org/10.1080/08927936.2016.1181364

Binfet, J. T., Passmore, H. A., Cebry, A., Struik, K., & McKay, C. (2018). Reducing university students' stress through a drop-in canine-therapy program. *Journal of Mental Health, 27*(3), 197–204. https://doi.org/10.1080/09638237.2017.1417551

BioKIDS. (n.d.). Kids' inquiry of diverse species: Giant African snail – Achatina Fulica. www.biokids.umich.edu/critters/Achatina_fulica/

Boss, L., Branson, S., Hagan, H., & Krause-Parello, C. (2019). A systematic review of equine-assisted interventions in military veterans diagnosed with PTSD. *Journal of Veterans Studies, 5*(1), 23–33. http://doi/org/10.21061/jvs.v5i1.134

Brelsford, V. L., Meints, K., Gee, N. R., & Pfeffer, K. (2017). Animal-assisted interventions in the classroom: A systematic review. *International Journal of Environmental Research and Public Health, 14*(7), 669.

Casey, J., Csiernik, R., Knezevic, D., & Ebear, J. (2017). The impact of animal-assisted interventions on staff in a senior residential care facility. *International Journal of Mental Health and Addiction, 16*, 1238–1248. https://doi.org/10.1007/s11469-017-9849-5

Chan, M., Schonert-Reichl, K. A., & Binfet, J. T. (2022). Human-animal interactions and the promotion of social and emotional competencies: A scoping review. *Anthrozoos, 35*(5), 647–692. https://doi.org/10.1080/08927936.2022.2042080

Colarelli, S. M., McDonald, A. M., Christensen, M. S., & Honts, C. (2017). A companion dog increases prosocial behavior in work groups. *Anthrozoös, 30*(1), 77–89. https://doi.org/10.1080.08927936.2017.1270595

Cooke, B., & Farrington, D. P. (2016). The effectiveness of dog-training programs in prison. *The Prison Journal, 96*(6), 1–23. https://doi.org/10.1177/0032885516671919

Crossman, M. K., Kazdin, A. E., & Knudson, K. (2015). Brief unstructured interaction with a dog reduces distress. *Anthrozoös, 28*(4), 649–659. https://doi.org/10.1080.08927936.2015

Deaton, C. (2005). Humanizing prisons with animals: A closer look at "cell dogs" and horse programs in correctional institutions. *Journal of Correctional Education, 56*(1), 46–62. www.jstor.org/stable/23282783

Dell, C., Williamson, L., McKenzie, H., Carey, B., Cruz, M., Gibson, M., & Pavelich, A. (2021). A commentary about lessons learned: Transitioning a therapy dog program online during the Covid-19 pandemic. *Animals, 11*, 914. https://doi.org/10.3390/ani11030914

Dodd, A. L., Priestly, M., Tyrrell, K., Cygan, S., Newell, C., & Byrom, N. C. (2021). University student well-being in the United Kingdom: A scoping review of its conceptualisation and measurement. Journal of Mental Health, *30*, 375–387. https://doi.org/10.1080/09638237.2021.1875419

Esteves, S., & Stokes, T. (2008). Social effects of a dog's presence on children with disabilities. *Anthrozoös, 21*(1), 5–15. https://doi.org/10.2752/089279308X274029

Fine, A. H., Tedeshi, P., & Elvove, E. (2015). Forward thinking: The evolving field of human-animal interactions. In A. H. Fine (Ed.), *Handbook on animal-assisted therapy: Foundations and guidelines for animal-assisted interventions* (pp. 21–35). Elsevier Academic Press. https://doi.org/10.1016/B978-0-12-801292-5.00003-1

Foerder, P., & Royer, M. (2021). The effect of therapy dogs on preoperative anxiety. *Anthrozoös, 34*(5), 659–670. https://doi.org/10.1080/08927936.2021.1914440

Fournier, A. K. (2019). *Animal-assisted intervention: Thinking empirically.* Palgrave MacMillian.

Hall, S., Gee, N. R., & Mills, D. S. (2016). Children reading to dogs: A systematic review of the literature. *PLoS ONE, 11*(2), E0149759 https://doi.org/10.1371/journal.pone.0149759

Harada, T., Ishizaki, F., Nitta, Y., Miki, Y., Numamoto, H., . . . Kohsaku, N. (2019). Relationship between the characteristics of therapy goats and children and older people. *International Medical Journal, 26*(5), 405–408.

Haraway, D. J. (2008). *When species meet.* University of Minnesota Press.

Harris, N. M., & Binfet, J. T. (2022). Exploring children's perceptions of an after-school canine-assisted social and emotional learning program: A case study. *Journal of Research in Childhood Education, 36*(1), 78–95. https://doi.org/10.1080/025685543.2020.1846643

Hartwig, E., & Binfet, J. T. (2019). What's important in canine-assisted intervention teams? An investigation of canine-assisted intervention program online screening tools. *Journal of Veterinary Behavior: Clinical Applications and Research, 29*, 53–60.

Hodgson, P., Cook, G., Johnson, A., & Abbott-Brailey, H. (2022). Ageing well with creative arts and pets: The HenPower story. *Activities, Adaptation & Aging.* https://doi.org/10.1080/10924788.2022.2116548

Huber, A., Klug, S. J., Abraham, A., Westenberg, E., Schmidt, V., & Winkler, A. S. (2022). Animal-assisted interventions improve mental, but not cognitive or physiological health outcomes of higher education students: A systematic review and meta-analysis. *International Journal of Mental Health and Addiction, 15*, 1–32. https://doi.org/10.1007/s11469-022-00945-4

Kazdin, A. E. (2017). Strategies to improve the evidence base of animal-assisted interventions. *Applied Developmental Science, 21*(2), 150–164. https://doi.org//10.1080/10888691.2016.1191952

Kingson, J. A. (2019, November 14). The llama as therapist. *New York Times.* www.nytimes.com/2019/11/14/well/live/llama-therapy-nursing-homes-elderly-seniors-hospitals-pet-therapy.html

Kinney, A. R., Eakman, A. M., Lassell, R., & Wood, W. (2019). Equine-assisted intervention for veterans with service-related health conditions: A systematic mapping review. *Military Medical Research, 6*(28), 1–15. https://doi.org/10.1186/s40779-019-0217-6

Kirnan, J. S., Siminerio, S., & Wong, Z. (2016). The impact of a therapy dog program on children's reading skills and attitudes toward reading. *Early Childhood Education Journal, 44*(6), 637–651. https://doi.org/10.1007/s10643-015-0747-9

Lobato Rincón, L. L., Rivera Martin, B., Medina Sanchez, M. A., Villafaina, S., Merellano-Navarro, E., & Collado-Mateo, D. (2021). Effects of dog-assisted education on physical and communicative skills in children with severe and multiple disabilities: A pilot study. *Animals, 11*(6), 1741. https://doi.org/10.2290/ani11061741

Matsuoka, A. K., & Sorenson, J. (2018). *Critical animal studies: Towards trans-species social justice.* Rowman & Littlefield International.

McNicholas, J., & Collis, G. M. (2000). Dogs as catalysts for social interactions: Robustness of the effect. *British Journal of Psychology, 91*, 61–70. https://doi.org/10.1348/000712600161673

Meints, K., Brelsford, V. L., Maréchal, L., Pennington, K., Rown, E., & Gee, N. R. (2022). Can dogs reduce stress levels in school children? Effects of dog-assisted interventions on salivary cortisol in children with and without special educational needs using randomized controlled trials. *PLoS ONE, 17*(6), e0269333. htttps://doi.org/10.1371/journal.pone.0269333

Molnár, M., Iváncsik, R., DiBlasio, B., & Nagy, I. (2020). Examining the effects of rabbit-assisted interventions in the classroom environment. *Animals, 10*(1), 26. https://doi.org/10.3390/ani10010026

Muckle, J., & Lasikiewicz, N. (2017). An exploration of the benefits of animal-assisted activities in undergraduate students in Singapore. *Asian Journal of School Psychology, 20*(2), 75–84. https://doi.org/10.1111/ajsp.12166

Mueller, M. K., Anderson, E. C., King, E. K., & Urry, H. L. (2021). Null effects of therapy dog interaction on adolescent anxiety during a laboratory-based social evaluative stressor. *Anxiety, Stress, & Coping: An International Journal, 34*(4), 365–380. https://doi.org/10.1080/10615806.2021.1892084

Mukherjee, U. (2020). Caring, relating, and becoming: Child-horse relationships in equestrian leisure. *Journal of Childhood Studies, 45*(2), 85–97. https://doi.org/10.18357/jcs452202019741

O'Haire, M. E., McKenzie, S. J., McCune, S., & Slaughter, V. (2013). Effects of animal-assisted activities with guinea pigs in the primary school classroom. *Anthrozoös, 26*(3), 445–458. https://doi.org/10.2752/1752/175303713X13697429463835

Parbery-Clark, C., Lubamba, M., Tanner, L., & McColl, E. (2021). Animal-assisted interventions for the improvement of mental health outcomes in higher education students: A systematic review of randomised controlled trials. *International Journal of Environmental Research and Public Health, 18*, 10768. https://doi.org/10.3390/ijerph182010768

Pendry, P., Carr, A. M., Roeter, S. M., & Vandagriff, J. L. (2018). Experimental trial demonstrates effects of animal-assisted stress prevention program on college students' positive and negative emotion. *Human-Animal Interaction Bulletin, 6*(1), 81–97.

Pendry, P., & Vandagriff, J. L. (2019). Animal visitation program (AVP) reduces cortisol levels of university students: A randomized controlled trial. *AERA Open, 5*(2), 1–12. https://doi.org/10.1177/2332858419852592

Pidgeon, M. (2018). Moving between theory and practice within an Indigenous research paradigm. *Qualitative Research, 19*(4), 418–436. https://doi.org/10.1017/1468794118781380

Pidgeon, M., & Hardy Cox, D. (2002). Researching with Aboriginal peoples: Practices and principles. *Canadian Journal of Native Education, 26*(2), 96–106.

Pidgeon, M., & Riley, T. (2021). Understanding the application and use of Indigenous research methodologies in the Social Sciences by Indigenous and non-Indigenous scholars. *International Journal of Education Policy & Leadership, 17*(8). https://doi.org/10.22230/ijepl.2021v17n8a1065

Ratschen, E., Shoesmith, E., Shahab, L., Silva, K., Kale, D., Toner, P., Reeve, C., & Mills, D. S. (2020). Human-animal relationships and interactions during the Covid-19 lockdown phase in the UK: Investigating links with mental health and loneliness. *PLoS ONE, 15*(10), e0239307. https://doi.org/10.1371/journal.pone.0239307

Reilly, K. M., Adesope, O. O., & Erdman, P. (2020). The effects of dogs on learning: A meta-analysis. *Anthrozoos, 33*(3), 339–360. https://doi.org/10.1080/08927936.2020.1746523

Rodriguez, K. E., Green, F. L. L., Binfet, J. T., Townsend, L., & Gee, N. R. (2023). Complexities and considerations in conducting animal-assisted intervention research: A discussion of randomized controlled trials. *Human-Animal Interactions.* https://doi.org/10.1079/hai.2023.0004

Rodriguez, K. E., Herzog, H., & Gee, N. R. (2021). Variability in human-animal interaction research. *Frontiers in Veterinary Science, 7*(6), 1–9. https://doi.org/10.3389/fvets.2020.619600

Rousseau, C. X., & Tardif-Williams, C. Y. (2019). Turning the page for spot: The potential of therapy dogs to support reading motivation among young children. *Anthrozoös, 32*(5), 665–677.

Sandt, D. D. (2020). Effective implementation of animal assisted education interventions in the inclusive early childhood education classroom. *Early Childhood Education Journal, 48*, 103–115. https://doi.

org/10.1007/s10643-019-01000-zScheck, H., Williamson, L., & Dell, C. A. (2022). Understanding psychiatric patients' experiences of virtual animal-assisted therapy sessions during COVID-19 pandemic. *People and Animals: The International Journal of Research and Practice, 5*(1).

Shapiro, K. (2020). Human-animal studies: Remembering the past, celebrating the present, troubling the future. *Society and Animals, 28*(7), 797–833. https://doi.org/10.1163/15685306-bja10029

Steel, J. (2023). Reading to dogs in schools: A controlled feasibility study of an online reading to dogs intervention. *International Journal of Educational Research, 117*, 102117. https://doi.org/10.1016/j.ijer.2022.102117

Tardif-Williams, C. Y., & Bosacki, S. (2015). Evaluating the impact of a humane education summer camp program on school-aged children's relationships with companion animals. *Anthrozoös, 28*(4), 587–600.

Toshihide, H., Ishizaki, F., Nitta, Y., & Miki, Y. (2019). Relationship between the characteristics of goat therapy and children and older people. *International Medical Journal, 26*(5), 405–408.

Villafaina-Dominguez, B., Collado-Mateo, D., Merellano-Navarro, E., & Villafaina, S. (2020). Effects of dog-based animal-assisted interventions in prison population: A systematic review. *Animals, 10*(11), 2129. https://doi.org/10.3390/ani10112129

Wagner, C., Grob, C., & Hediger, K. (2022). Specific and non-specific factors of animal-assisted interventions considered in research: A systematic review. *Frontiers in Psychology*, 158103. https://www.crd.york.ac.uk/prospero/display_record.php?

Wijker, C., van der Steen, S., Spek, A., Leontjevas, R., & Enders-Slegers, M. J. (2020). Social development of adults with autism spectrum disorder during dog-assisted therapy: A detailed observational analysis. *International Journal of Environment of Research in Public Health, 17*(16), 5922. https://doi.org/10.3390/ijerph17165922

Wilson, E. O. (1984). *Biophilia*. Harvard University Press.

World Health Organization. (2023). Health and wellbeing. www.who.int/data/gho/data/major-themes/health-and-well-being

3 Exploring Asynchronous and Synchronous Opportunities for Virtual Human-Animal Interactions

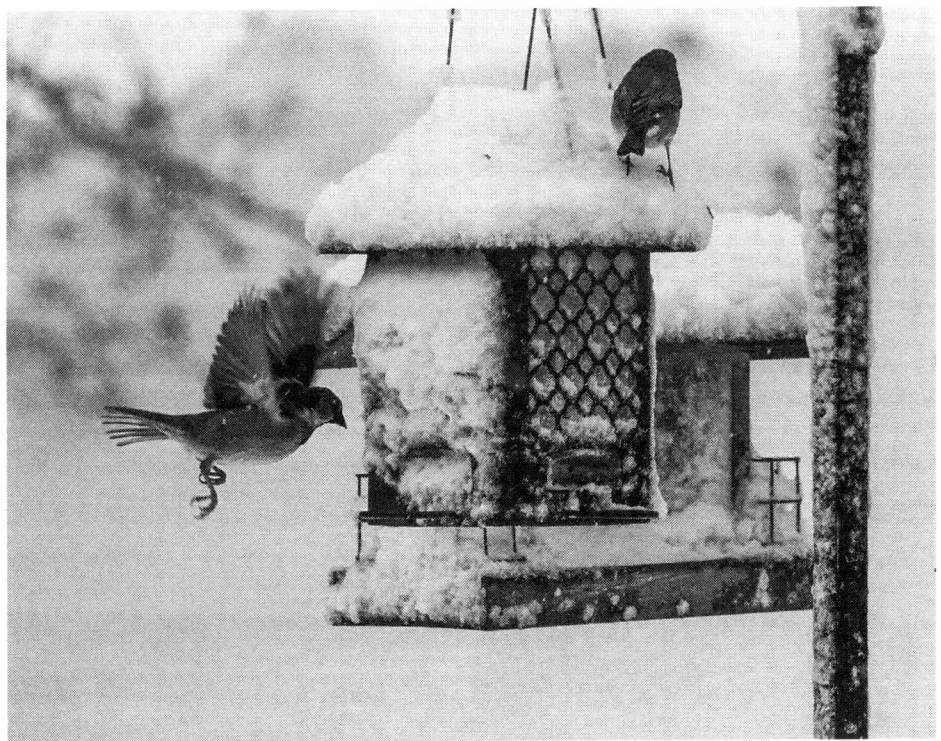

Figure 3.1 Birds at feeder provide joy to viewers

Source: Pixabay

Scenario

I had no idea birds could be watched this way!

Pat had long enjoyed having a bird feeder at her family home. Now, as a senior living in a communal care facility, she found herself unable to have a bird feeder and watch her favourite birds enjoy the buffet she'd put out daily. Pat was a fan of watching YouTube videos of birds at feeders, but when her daughter suggested watching birds visiting feeders in real time on her iPad, she was thrilled. It brought her right back to being at her kitchen window and

DOI: 10.4324/9781003327868-3

watching cardinals cracking seeds and the territorial song birds defend their feeding station. She marvelled at how some people were so trusted that they could even feed wild birds from their hand. Pat sometimes needed help in finding the link to the livestream on her iPad, but once she did, she'd often proclaim that watching the bird feeder livestream calmed her and was the highlight of her day. In fact, her daughter would often call and start their conversation with "Okay, what did the cardinals do today?"

Questions for Reflection

1. What might a livestream of birds at the feeder provide that YouTube videos don't?
2. What livestream opportunities are there for humans to observe animals?
3. Do synchronous virtual connections engage viewers to a greater extent over asynchronous viewings?
4. What benefits might arise from synchronous and asynchronous animal observations?
5. Can people establish and nurture bonds with animals virtually?
6. Can virtual human-animal interactions connect people to other people?

Our last chapter provided an overview of human-animal interaction (HAI) research including considerations for determining the rigour or value of published research examining the effects of interacting with animals on human well-being. The aim of the current chapter is to examine the different ways that humans might interact virtually with animals and provide an overview of both asynchronous and synchronous opportunities to establish virtual human-animal connections. Our chapter begins with an overview of common virtual pathways to bolstering well-being and concludes with an overview of the emerging research attesting to the benefits of spending virtual time with animals.

Our opening scenario in which a senior citizen in a care facility derives joy from both asynchronous (i.e., viewing static YouTube videos) and synchronous (i.e., livestream bird feeder

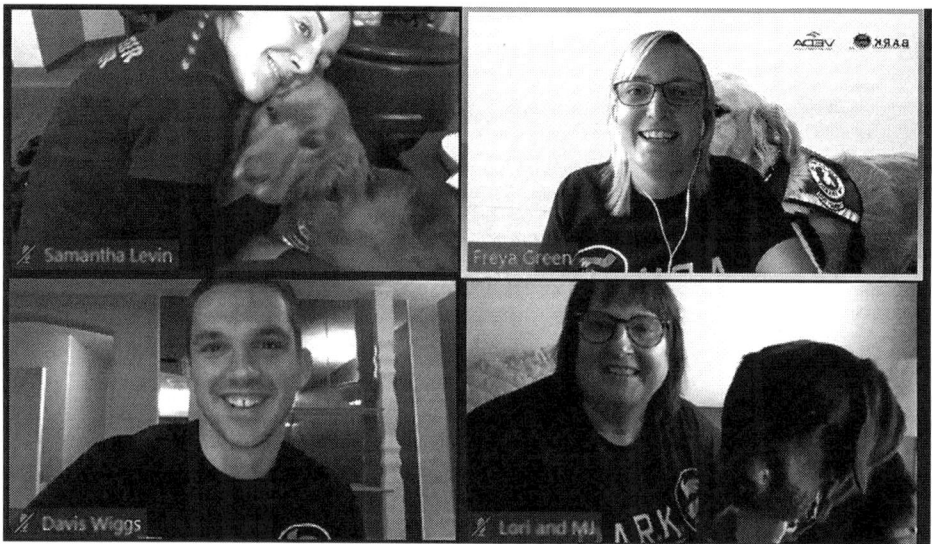

Figure 3.2 Zoom session with students and therapy dogs

Source: F. L. L. Green Photography

viewing) virtual observations of birds at a feeder illustrates the variability in opportunities for humans to connect virtually with animals. Accustomed to viewing YouTube videos, Pat was unaware of the option of viewing a live feed (video transmitted in actual time) to watch birds at a feeder. Upon discovering the livestream option, the opportunity for Pat to spend time connecting with animals was both enriched and expanded.

Why Virtual Human-Animal Interactions Are Needed and Important

As we introduced in Chapter 1, providing virtual opportunities for individuals to interact with animals is important for a number of reasons. First, there has been increased isolation arising from Covid-19 that saw a significant decrease in opportunities for humans to interact with one another. This isolation, in turn, has contributed to a whole host of negative outcomes including depression and a sense of loneliness (Thomas et al., 2022). Second, it has been argued that Covid-19 restrictions exacerbated underlying or preexisting mental health challenges. That is, what was once manageable and did not significantly impede one's quality of life was rendered challenging and sometimes impaired optimal functioning. Third, nascent research on the effects of VHAIs suggests that connecting with animals in a virtual context is a viable way to bolster well-being benefits in humans and may provide an inexpensive and accessible way for humans to connect with animals. In fact, it might be considered an easily accessed and low-barrier well-being resource. Fourth, asynchronous virtual content may be accessed by humans at the time they need it. There is no scheduling of appointments or waiting in queue to access virtual animal content. In this regard, this resource is at the beck and call of the humans seeking to bolster their well-being (i.e., real-time support). Robino and colleagues (2022) have recently written on the effects of animal-assisted crisis response to reduce the stress of school shooting survivors. Within the realm of psychological first aid, we typically see animal-assisted crisis response teams travel to sites to offer in-person support. Imagine that while teams are travelling, virtual support could be immediately offered to those in need. Last, the offering of virtual animal content to bolster well-being might be especially appealing to those humans who are reluctant to seek help. As accessing virtual animal content is considered low-barrier (i.e., no preregistration, free to access), humans who are reticent about seeking help may be more willing to access asynchronous modules. In this regard, virtual animal content may serve as an initial step in establishing a well-being regime or protocol and may possibly serve as a catalyst for humans to seek additional synchronous support.

> Within the mental health professions, the model of delivering psychosocial interventions is expanding. Many of these involve the use of technology and online versions of treatment that draw on the internet and other media, including video, phone, and application software (apps) for smartphones and tablets.
>
> (Kazdin & Rabbit, 2013, p. 172)

Providing Virtual Access to Support Individuals With Phobias or Allergies

In addition to the advantages reviewed previously that arise when humans are provided with virtual opportunities to connect with animals, we see distinct and unique advantages for individuals with either phobias or allergies that impede or prevent them from interacting in-person with animals. The prevalence of animal phobias ranges between 3.3% to 7%, and animal phobias remain one of the more prevalent types of social phobias (Botella et al., 2016). Few people with phobias seek treatment, and it has been posited that a lack of treatments addressing specific phobias undergirds this lack of help-seeking but also that long waiting lists to access experienced counsellors are a deterrent (Kazdin, 2014). We submit that virtual human-animal connections may provide an opportunity for individuals seeking support to overcome their fear of animals.

VHAIs may also provide opportunities for individuals suffering from allergies to establish meaningful connections with animals. It is estimated that 10% to 20% of the world's population suffer from allergies to companion dogs and cats (Chan & Leung, 2018). This, in turn, restricts these individuals' abilities to interact in-person with animals. Engaging with either synchronous or asynchronous virtual animal content is a possible pathway through which these individuals, especially children, might participate in HAIs.

Providing Virtual Access to Support Children and Families Unable to Have Pets

Recall the opening scenario in Chapter 1 in which Megan pleads with her mom to get a kitten but this is not feasible because her sister, Amanda, is allergic to cats. Just as animal phobias can restrict opportunities for HAI, there may be situations where children yearn to have a family companion animal, and for a variety of reasons, the parents or guardians are unable to incorporate one into their family. It could be due to one member of the family having an allergy or a phobia, but it could also be because of housing, cultural, or financial reasons. Increasingly, we find ourselves living in high-density, urban housing that can make having companion animals a challenge. Having companion animals can be forbidden by rental regulations or space restrictions, for example. It's also important to recognize the respective role of animals within different cultures. Cultural perspectives on animals might position animals as living outdoors and as insufficiently clean to share indoor living spaces with humans. Last, it is important to recognize that having family companion animals is increasingly an expensive undertaking. The husbandry related to keeping a companion dog, for example, as estimated by the Ontario Veterinary Medical Association (2021), hovers near $4,000. There are, thus, financial considerations that restrict families' abilities to welcome a companion animal into their home and this, in turn, positions virtual connections with companion animals as one possible and appealing way for families to address barriers around phobias, allergies, or finances.

Virtual Opportunities Supporting Well-Being

We are increasingly living in a digital world and the incorporation of technology into our day-to-day activities has especially increased access to services for people living in remote or under-resourced areas. As illustrated by the scenario at the outset of Chapter 2, in which Jacob who is a college student living his life almost entirely online was perplexed by not having virtual access to therapy dogs, tasks that were only uniquely available to us in-person may now be accomplished or accessed via digital means. Illustrations of this transition from in-person to virtual tasks abound, and we now regularly shop and visit others through screens, when historically these things were done uniquely in-person.

For some time now, virtual opportunities have been available for individuals seeking to bolster their well-being. This next section explores the various iterations of virtual well-being support available and lays the foundation for our later discussion of virtual pathways for human-animal interactions. Hazma and colleagues (2021, p. 2) have argued that Covid-19 has exacerbated public well-being and support the claim that increased access to virtual well-being and mental health support is looming.

Many have suggested that mental health concerns will increase globally in response to the pandemic (Gunnell et al., 2020; Holmes et al., 2020), and some have even argued that the psychological impacts will be as significant as the physical health impacts from COVID-19, particularly for vulnerable populations (Galea et al., 2020; Ornell et al., 2020).

Within a formal counselling framework, virtual therapy has emerged as a way of offering support to clients and can take one of two forms: (1) asynchronous, self-directed access to programs that see clients follow modules that might present them with information and a series of exercises (e.g., breathing) to complete; and (2) synchronous access to a therapist that might see a therapist and client meet virtually in real-time for a session.

Acknowledging the Role of Animal-Assisted Interventions as an Adjunct Intervention

We recognize that AAIs aimed at reducing stress and, more broadly, boosting well-being are considered adjunct interventions. They are not intended to be a primary source of mental health support but rather one that can serve as a catalyst for clients to seek additional, more formal modes of support (i.e., one-on-one counselling). Here we distinguish AAIs from the field of animal-assisted therapy or counselling that requires advanced training on the part of the therapist and delivers frontline therapeutic interventions to clients. As an illustration of the training required by therapists who, as part of their professional practice, collaborate with animals, readers are invited to investigate the program offered by Dr. Elizabeth Hartwig of Texas State University, who is the Director of the Texas State University Animal-Assisted Counselling (AAC) Academy (Texas State University, n.d.). Described as "a professional training program that promotes the human-animal bond through the study and practice of animal-assisted counseling" (p. 1), Hartwig's work advances counsellors' capacities to enrich the therapeutic experience by working alongside therapy animals.

Returning to AAIs, in our emerging research examining the effects of virtual canine comfort sessions (see Binfet et al., 2022, p. 4), we describe canine-assisted interventions as "a complimentary therapeutic approach – not intended to stand on their own as a comprehensive treatment but rather to offer support to clients in addition to other available services (Marcus, 2013; Nepps et al., 2014; Nimer & Lundahl, 2007; Rossetti & King, 2010)." Again, within the context of on-campus canine visitation programs, Pendry and colleagues (2021) postulate that such programs may be especially appealing to individuals who eschew other, more traditional or formal, avenues of seeking help and support. We, thus, position virtual human-animal connections as one possible well-being resource that people can access that might provide temporary support, and this support may, in turn, render these individuals to be more receptive to, and possibly seek out, more formal sources of support.

Empirical Work Attesting to the Efficacy of Virtual Human-Animal Interactions

Forging new empirical terrain is HAI researcher Colleen Dell from the University of Saskatchewan who, along with colleagues (2021), offered initial insights into transitioning an in-person therapy dog program to a virtual context. Within the context of an on-campus AAI implemented to support college students' well-being, Dell and colleagues chronicle their pathway to adapting a previously in-person AAI to a virtual context. Several key findings from their commentary illuminate our understanding of the nuances or mechanisms requiring consideration. First, making use of existing social media platforms was a strategic first step to ensure that the virtual content was "meeting individuals where they are at, so they can view the content at their convenience" (Dell et al., 2021, p. 4) and to ensure that content was delivered in a format familiar to viewers. The use of social media also afforded opportunities for viewers to engage with the content by posing questions or comments. Social media also served as a platform through which the virtual programming could be advertised. With regards to the content of the AAIs, Dell and colleagues showcased a variety of interactions that included taking a dog for a walk, participating in a healthy food taste test, therapy dog training, grooming, taking photos, and a tutorial on dog skin care. On average, virtual content was presented in 15-minute segments and was offered via live or prerecorded formats.

A key lesson arising from the transition from in-person to a virtual format revealed that dog handlers required support as they adapted to a virtual context. Dell and colleagues (2021) note that some of the handlers were reluctant of the permanent nature of the online videos they'd be creating. Relatedly, the handlers required additional information and training to help them adjust to the virtual context, especially around technical aspects of filming (e.g., minimizing background noise reduction). With respect to the therapy dogs themselves, handlers required support in how best to involve their therapy dog during the online sessions. Establishing a routine helped the dogs interact naturally in front of the camera. With regards to the information shared, handlers offered mental health tips and drew from a handler handbook to assist their supporting viewers' mental well-being. Thus, we see ample structure in the work presented here both in the routine to render the therapy dogs at ease during online sessions and to help guide the handlers in their sharing of information with viewers. The culmination of these efforts resulted in a repository of videos on YouTube that could be accessed by viewers far and wide.

The insights of Dell and colleagues (2021) offer an initial foray into virtual AAIs, and although these authors administered a needs assessment questionnaire, no pre-to-post effects of their VHAIs were determined. Extending the work of Dell and colleagues, we set out to empirically assess the effects of virtual canine comfort modules on undergraduate student well-being. Next, we review the first (to our knowledge) randomized controlled trial to answer the question: Does spending time virtually with therapy dogs reduce stress?

Recently published in the journal *Anthrozoös,* our research saw 467 undergraduate students (primarily first- and second-year students) provide informed consent and complete a series of self-report well-being measures (e.g., stress, anxiety, positive and negative affect, loneliness, connectedness to others) (Binfet et al., 2022). To tease apart the effects of both live versus prerecorded and dog or no-dog conditions, we then randomly assigned participants to one of the four conditions described in Table 3.1. In Chapter 2, we discussed the variability in intervention duration, and this study employed a 5-minute intervention and, in this way, would certainly be considered on the brief end of the duration spectrum. A brief intervention was purposefully chosen as we wanted to test whether abbreviated "canine comfort modules" might offer well-being support, thus establishing that even briefly accessed VHAI offers benefits.

It merits noting here that the dog-handler teams were all experienced veterans of the B.A.R.K. program and attended an orientation session to familiarize both the dogs and the handlers with the studio in which filming took place. To ensure consistency across the conditions, the handlers followed a script that was designed to mirror, as closely as possible, a typical dialogue that might occur in an on-campus CAI. The findings revealed that regardless of the intervention to which participants were assigned, participants reported feeling more positive emotional states (see Figures 3.4 and 3.5); less stressed, anxious, and lonely; a decrease in

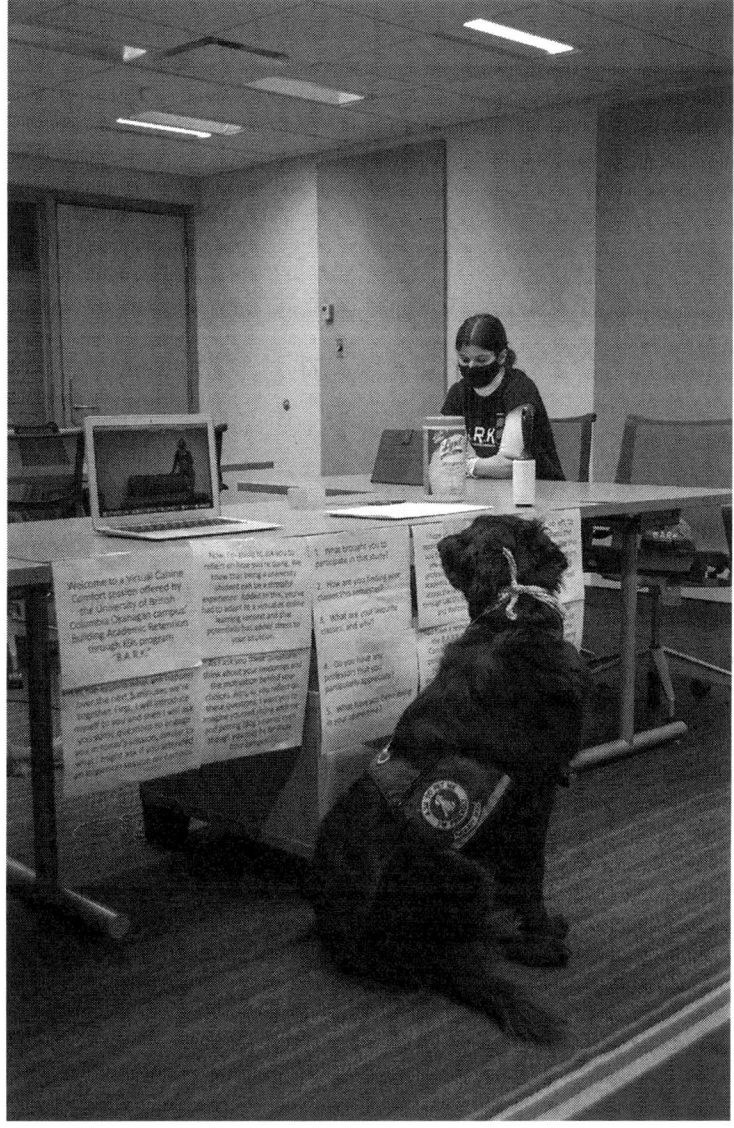

Figure 3.3 Therapy dog Punim waiting for virtual session to begin

Source: F. L. L. Green Photography

Table 3.1 Conditions Across Synchronous and Asynchronous Dog and No-Dog Conditions

Condition	Synchronous	Asynchronous
Treatment	Live Virtual Canine Comfort Module with a dog-handler team delivered via Zoom. Handlers to follow a script.	Prerecorded Virtual Canine Comfort Module with a dog-handler team delivered via YouTube. Handlers to follow a script.
Control	Live handler-only condition delivered via Zoom. Handlers to follow a script.	Prerecorded handler-only condition delivered via YouTube. Handlers to follow a script.

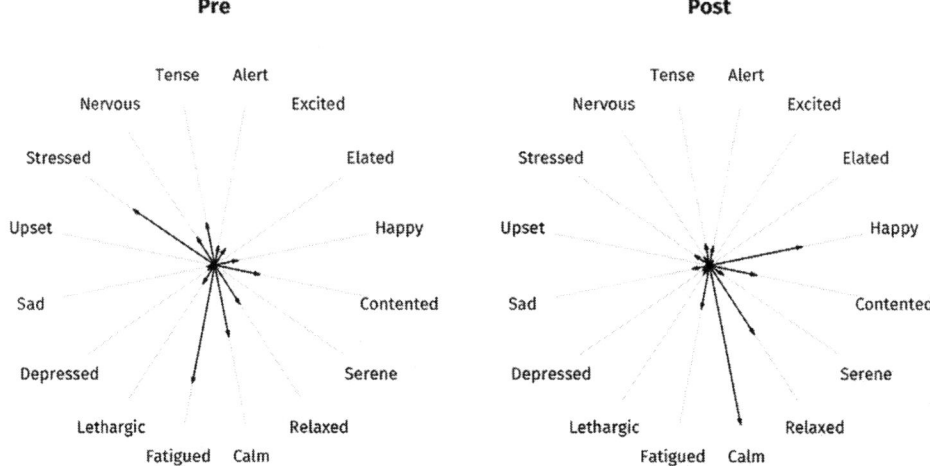

Figure 3.4 Pre- and post-descriptors of emotion across groups

Source: reprinted with permission from *Anthrozoös*

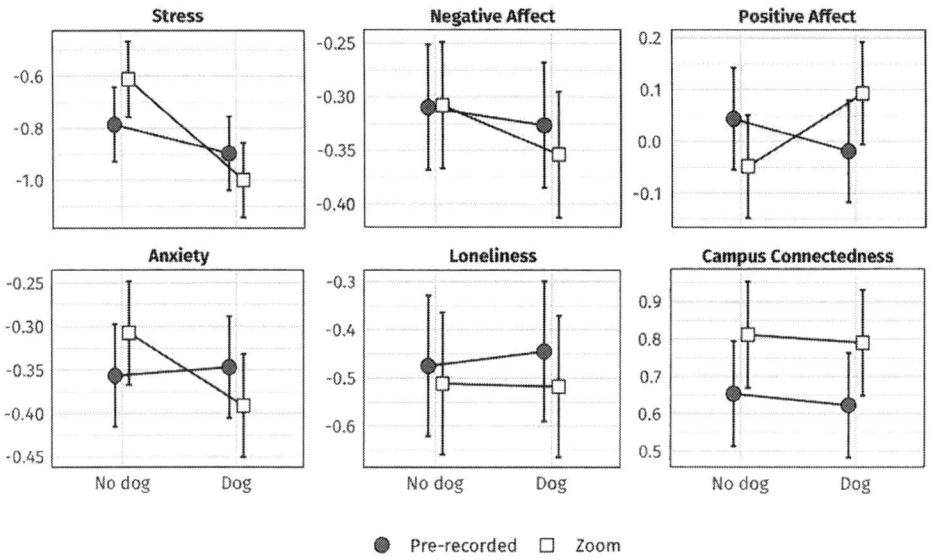

Figure 3.5 Therapy dog versus no dog pre-to-post-test changes on outcome variables

Source: reprinted with permission from *Anthrozoös*

their self-report of negative affect; and a stronger sense of connectedness. Examining the dog versus no-dog conditions revealed that the presence of a dog was associated with greater self-reports of stress reduction, regardless of whether participants were in synchronous (Zoom) or asynchronous (prerecorded videos) conditions. Contrary to our hypothesis, we did not find any superadditive effects whereby participants in the Zoom + dog condition reported significant boosts to well-being. Although additional research is needed, the implications of our first empirical foray into assessing the effects of virtual canine comfort modules helps us understand that virtual CAI, regardless of whether the dog is presented synchronously (live on camera) or asynchronously (via a prerecorded video), bolsters the viewers' overall well-being and contributes to a significant reduction in self-reports of pre-to-post viewing stress. These findings are in concert with the findings of in-person research attesting to the benefits of spending time in-person with therapy dog-handler teams (Barker et al., 2016; Binfet et al., 2018; Pendry et al., 2018).

As part of our randomized controlled trial study, we also sought to forge new empirical terrain by qualitatively exploring students' insights and perceptions about *why* spending time virtually with therapy dogs reduces stress. In this case, participants were asked to share their views of their experience by rating statements and responding to open-ended prompts. These findings were recently published in *People and Animals: International Journal of Research and Practice* (Tardif-Williams et al., 2023), and thematic content analysis of findings revealed that, in addition to the therapy dogs, type of delivery was also related to students' well-being experiences. For instance, overall, participants in the synchronous condition with a dog reported more favorable well-being benefits as compared with participants in the asynchronous condition with a dog. Notably, a sense of feeling *comforted/supported* was most likely to be identified by participants in the synchronous condition with a dog compared to the asynchronous condition with a dog. It is possible that the presence of the therapy dog in the synchronous condition might have acted as a social catalyst, helping to unite participants virtually. In this way, some students might be drawn to virtual CAIs as a way to promote group or collaborative activities. In addition, our intervention design requiring participants to always show their faces during synchronous sessions (versus turning their camera off as is commonplace during typical virtual sessions for university students), likely helped foster this sense of community. Finally, it is worth noting that in our study the participants in the asynchronous session with a dog present still reported well-being benefits but seemingly for different reasons. Specifically, the participants shared that the prerecorded sessions with a dog allowed them to be more mindful and to reflect in a quiet space about the things that mattered to them. These findings attest to the notion that participants may respond and engage differently to virtual human-animal connections for different reasons. We return to the topics of mindfulness and individual differences in Chapter 6 when we discuss best practices for creating and delivering and engaging people in virtual human-animal connections.

Also informing our understanding of how virtual HAI might support the well-being of clients is found in the recent research of Scheck and colleagues (2022), who transitioned an in-person canine-assisted therapy program to a virtual format to support incarcerated individuals needing mental health support. Using a case study methodology of four patients, semi-structured interviews were used to explore participants' perceptions of the virtual format, the role of the handler, and their perceptions of the support they received (i.e., emotional support and feelings of hope, normalcy, and deinstitutionalization). These authors recognize the need for additional research to assess the effects of virtual canine-assisted therapy; however, their findings inform our understanding of how connections may be established between clients and dog-handler teams and how dog-handler teams are perceived as a key source of emotional support – even when available virtually. Further, we note that the unique insights generated by qualitative research conducted by Dell and colleagues (2021), Scheck and colleagues (2022), and Tardif-Williams and colleagues (2023) respond to recent calls for more qualitatively focused research in the field of HAIs and meaningfully inform the creation and delivery of opportunities for virtual human-animal connections, a topic that we discuss further in Chapter 6.

Conclusion

The aim of this chapter was to provide an overview of the nascent field of research examining the viability of providing VHAIs as a means of supporting learning, social connections, and enhancing human well-being. Emerging research findings attest to the potential of virtual opportunities for HAIs to provide support to varied human clients and elicit favourable well-being outcomes, notably around stress reduction. We recognized in this chapter the restricted reach of AAIs (including VHAIs), noting that they are an adjunct or complimentary form of support not intended to replace formal counselling or therapy. Delving further into opportunities for humans to virtually connect with animals, our next chapter provides an in-depth overview of the role that social media plays in affording human-animal connections.

References

Barker, S. B., Barker, R. T., McCain, N. L., & Schubert, C. M. (2016). A randomized cross-over exploratory study of the effect of visiting therapy dogs on college student stress before final exams. *Anthrozoös, 29*, 35–46. https://doi.org/10.1080/08927936.2015.1069988

Binfet, J. T., Passmore, H. A., Cebry, A., Struik, K., & McKay, C. (2018). Reducing university students' stress through a drop-in canine-therapy program. *Journal of Mental Health, 3*, 197–204. https://doi.org/10.1080/09638237.2017.1417551

Binfet, J. T., Tardif-Williams, C., Draper, Z. A., Green, F. L. L., Singal, A., Rousseau, C. X., & Roma, R. (2022). Virtual canine comfort: A randomized controlled trial of the effects of a canine-assisted intervention supporting undergraduate wellbeing. *Anthrozoös, 35*(6), 809–832. https://doi.org/10.1080/08927936.2022.2062866

Botella, C., Pérez-Ara, M. A., Bretón-López, J., Quero, S., Garcia-Palacios, A., & Banos, R. M. (2016). In vivo versus augmented reality exposure in the treatment of small animal phobia: A randomized controlled trial. *PLoS One, 11*(2), e0148237. https://doi.org/10.1371/journal.pone.0148237

Chan, S. K., & Leung, D. Y. M. (2018). Dog and cat allergies: Current state of diagnostic approaches and challenges. Allergy Asthma Immunology Research, 10(2), 97–105. https://doi.org/10.4168/aair.2018.10.2.97

Dell, C., Williamson, L., McKenzie, H., Carey, B., Cruz, M., Gibson, M., & Pavelich, A. (2021). A commentary about lessons learned: Transitioning a therapy dog program online during the Covid-19 pandemic. *Animals, 11*, 914. https://doi.org/10.3390/ani11030914

Galea, S., Merchant, R. M., & Lurie, N. (2020). The mental health consequences of COVID-19 and physical distancing. *Journal of the American Medical Association, 180,* 817–818. http://dx.doi.org/10.1002/da.20838

Gunnell, D., Appleby, L., Arensman, E., Hawton, K., John, A., . . . Pirkis, J. (2020). Suicide risk and prevention during the COVID-19 pandemic. *The Lancet Psychiatry, 7,* 468–471. https://doi.org/10.1016/S2215-0366(20)30171-1

Hamza, C. A., Ewing, L., Heath, N. L., & Goldstein, A. L. (2021). When social isolation is nothing new: A longitudinal study on psychological distress during COVID-19 among university students with and without preexisting mental health concerns. *Canadian Psychology/Psychologie Canadienne, 62*(1), 20–30. https://doi.org/10.1037/cap0000255

Holmes, E. A., O'Connor, R. C., Perry, V. H., Tracey, I., Wessely, S., . . . Arseneault, L. (2020). Multidisciplinary research priorities for the COVID-19 pandemic: A call for action for mental health science. *The Lancet Psychiatry, 7,* 547–560. http://dx.doi.org/10.1016/S2215-0366(20)30168-1

Kazdin, A. E. (2014). Evidence-based psychotherapies II: Changes in models of treatment and treatment deliveries. *South African Journal of Psychology, 45*(1), 3–21. https://doi.org/10.1177/008124631458733

Kazdin, A. E., & Rabbit, S. M. (2013). Novel models for delivering mental health services and reducing the burdens of mental illness. *Clinical Psychological Science, 1*(2), 170–191. https://doi.org/10.1177/2167702612463566

Marcus, D. A. (2013). The science behind animal-assisted therapy. *Current Pain and Headache Reports, 17,* 322. https://doi.org/10.1007/s11916-013-0322-2

Nepps, P., Stewart, C. N., & Bruckno, S. R. (2014). Animal-assisted activity: Effects of a complementary intervention program on psychological and physiological variables. *Journal of Evidence-Based Complementary & Alternative Medicine, 19,* 211–215. https://doi.org/10.1177/2156587214533570

Nimer, J., & Lundahl, B. (2007). Animal-assisted therapy: A meta-analysis. *Anthrozoös, 20,* 225–238. https://doi.org/10.2752/089279307X224773

Ontario Veterinary Medical Association. (2021). *The annual cost of owning a dog.* www.ovma.org/assets/1/6/CostOfCare%202021%20Canine.pdf

Ornell, F., Schuch, J. B., Sordi, A. O., & Kessler, F. H. P. (2020). "Pandemic fear" and COVID-19: Mental health burden and strategies. *Revista brasileira de psiquiatria, 42,* 232–235. http://dx.doi.org/10.1590/1516-4446-2020-0008

Pendry, P., Carr, A. M., Roeter, S. M., & Vandagriff, J. L. (2018). Experimental trial demonstrates effects of animal-assisted stress prevention program on college students' positive and negative emotion. *Human-Animal Interaction Bulletin, 6*(1), 81–97.

Pendry, P., Carr, A. M., Vandagriff, J. L., & Gee, N. R. (2021). Incorporating human-animal interaction into academic stress management programs: Effects on typical and at-risk college students' executive function. *AERA Open, 7*(1), 1–18. https://journals.sagepub.com/home/ero

Robino, A. E., Feldman, D. M., Stein, A. N., Schmaltz, M. A., Fitzpatrick, H. A., . . . Feldman, O. (2022). Sustained effects of animal-assisted crisis response on stress in school shooting survivors. *Human Animal Interaction Bulletin, 12*(2), 65–85. https://doi.org/10.1079/hai.2022.0019

Rossetti, J., & King, C. (2010). Animal-assisted therapy with psychiatric patients. *Journal of Psychosocial Nursing, 48,* 45–48. doi: 10.3928/02793695-20100831-05

Scheck, H., Williamson, L., & Dell, C. A. (2022). Understanding psychiatric patients' experiences of virtual animal-assisted therapy sessions during COVID-19 pandemic. *People and Animals: The International Journal of Research and Practice, 5*(1).

Tardif-Williams, C. Y., Binfet, J. T., Green, F. L. L., Roma, R., Akshat, S., Rousseau, C. X., & Godard, R. J. (2023). When therapy dogs provide virtual comfort: Exploring university students' insights and perspectives. *People and Animals: The International Journal of Research and Practice, 6*(1), 1–17. https://docs.lib.purdue.edu/paij/vol6/iss1/5

Texas State University. (n.d.). Animal-Assisted Counseling (AAC) Academy. www.txst.edu/clas/Professional-Counseling/Program-Faculty/Elizabeth-Kjellstrand-Hartwig.html

Thomas, L. E., Emich, A., Weiss, E., Zisman, C., Foray, K., Roberts, D. M., Page, E., & Ernst, M. (2022). Examination of the COVID-19 pandemic's impact on mental health from three perspectives: Global, social, and individual. *Association for Psychological Science, 18*(2), 513–526. https://doi.org/10.1177/17456916221078310

4 The Unique Role of Social Media in Fostering Informal Virtual Human-Animal Connections

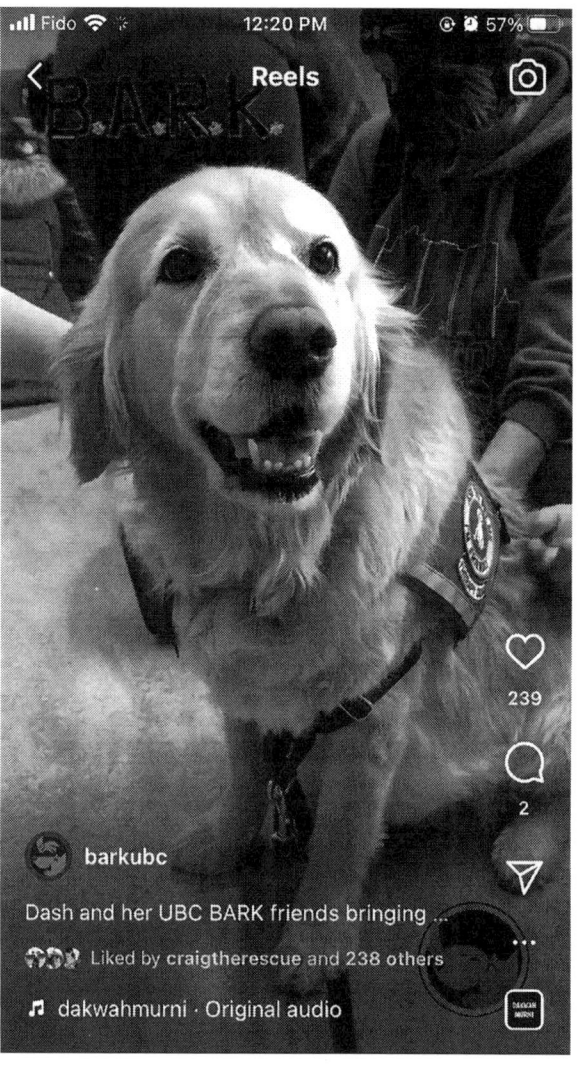

Figure 4.1 Instagram reel of students petting therapy dog Dash at UBC's B.A.R.K. program

Source: F. L. L. Green Photography

DOI: 10.4324/9781003327868-4

Scenario

All my friends have an Instagram account for their pets! I want to share fun pictures of my cat and dog with my friends.

Stefan has recently asked his parents if he can create an Instagram account to share pictures of their family dog and cat with his friends. He points out that all his friends share cute pictures of their pets on Instagram – it's a lot of fun! Stefan is 11 years old, but his parents think that he's still too young to create and maintain a social media account. They believe firmly that preteens should be discouraged from spending time on social media. They've heard about how some preteens can experience serious bullying and harassment on social media. Instead, they think that Stefan should be spending more time in nature and with his friends doing outdoor activities. However, Stefan's parents notice that he spends most of his time at home and indoors after school. They also recall a concern that his teacher raised at their last parent-teacher meeting. Stefan's teacher noted that he is experiencing challenges in making friends and that he does not always appear socially confident. Stefan's parents are now facing a dilemma, and they wonder if they should relax their stance on social media and grant Stefan permission to develop an Instagram account as it might help to increase his social confidence and facilitate friendships.

Questions for Reflection

1. What types of social media platforms are popular among children and adults?
2. What are some of the benefits and risks of social media for people's well-being?
3. Why and in what ways do people engage with animals on social media platforms?
4. Could having an Instagram account to share pictures of his dog and cat with his friends help increase Stefan's social confidence and enhance his friendships?

Social Media Platforms

Recent technological advances have revolutionized the way that people communicate with one another. The increased use of digital technologies such as computers, the internet, and social media platforms has expanded and transformed people's professional networking and their social networks. Social media involves the web and mobile platforms that facilitate social interactions within a virtual context or network (e.g., Facebook, YouTube, Instagram, TikTok, Twitter, Snapchat, VSCO). Using social media, people can connect with others to share and cocreate various forms of digital content including pictures, videos, and messages (Ahmed et al., 2019). In this way, new digital technologies along with social media have significantly reshaped features of people's social interactions and relationships. People can use both digital technologies and social media platforms to interact socially, and they can do this synchronously, in real time, or asynchronously, at an unscheduled time.

Today, unlike any other time in history, people have the means to connect and interact with a diverse group of people around the world as they explore their professional, social, and recreational interests. Recently, people's use of digital technologies and social media platforms has rapidly proliferated in response to the social constraints associated with the Covid-19 pandemic. In 2022, there were an estimated 4.62 billion social media users worldwide which represents half the global population (Hannahcurrey, 2022). Among younger users, 97% of adolescents between the ages of 13–17 report using the internet daily, and most report using at least one of the more popular social media platforms described in this section (Vogels et al., 2022). It is important to note that social media platforms shift rapidly along with trends in how people use these various platforms. Although the field of social media is ever evolving, we discuss some of the major social media platforms at the time of writing this book.

As might be expected, people's relationships with and affinity for all types of animals have also generalized into the digital world with animal-focused content proliferating on the internet and social media platforms (Rault, 2015). Indeed, images of dogs and cats figure prominently in the visual or "cute economy" of the internet (Meese, 2014). Social media allows people to share videos, pictures (including selfies with animals, animals taking selfies, and animal memes), descriptions and daily stories of their beloved companion animals, training tips, and information about healthy food options and treatment of common diseases. It also allows them to continuously monitor their companion animals' health and well-being and sustain their shared emotional connection when they are separated (via a remote pet camera); engage with virtual therapy animals; enjoy virtual visits to zoos, aquariums, animal sanctuaries, and wildlife centres; and engage in virtual social media challenges with their companion animals (e.g., *Call Your Dog Challenge*). In this way, by facilitating opportunities for social connection and creativity through animals, social media can be useful in bridging communities and fostering social connections among diverse people. People can use both digital technologies and social media platforms to showcase and share with others what they appreciate most about animals. In this chapter, we explore the unique role of social media in fostering informal VHAIs. We begin with a discussion of various existing social media platforms and the increasingly important role of social media in people's lives and note how people might engage differently with social media as a function of age and gender. We then explore the many ways that animals tend to feature prevalently within social media and discuss some of the ways that informal VHAIs might foster well-being among social media users. We conclude with a discussion about the importance of safeguarding animal welfare within digital or virtual human-animal contexts.

Facebook

Currently, Facebook is one of the most popular social media platforms with over 2.9 billion monthly active users (Omnicore Agency, 2022). Facebook is an online social media and social networking platform wherein users can create a profile to share information about themselves. People can post text, photos, or videos to be shared with any other people who have agreed to be their *friends*. Facebook also offers different privacy settings for people who wish to share their information more publicly. Also, people can communicate with each other directly through the Facebook Messenger platform, join social networking groups (e.g., Rescue Dogs Canada), and receive notifications on the activities of their Facebook *friends* and *selected groups*. In this way, Facebook helps people stay connected with one another (e.g., family, friends, work colleagues, acquaintances) and with their companion animals, meet new people and groups, and be a part of different communities. Today, Facebook users tend to be millennials or young adults ranging in age from 25–35 years. Still, 36% of Facebook users are aged 45 years or over. While a small percentage of teenagers (3.9%) has a Facebook account, these teenagers they tend not to use them as often (Barnhart, 2022). Across age categories, Facebook users tend to be equally distributed across gender (56% male, 44% female) and are located around the world with the largest base of active users located in countries such as India, the United States, Indonesia, Brazil, Mexico, and the Philippines. It merits noting that, due to its popularity among a diverse group of people, Facebook is still the most used platform among marketers (Omnicore Agency, 2022).

YouTube

YouTube is the second most popular social media platform with over 2.6 billion monthly active users (Omnicore Agency, 2022). YouTube is a video sharing website where users can easily create and share videos with others and watch online videos posted by others. YouTube pages can have *followers* and receive *likes*, thus increasing their popularity. In this way, YouTube also holds the possibility to facilitate online social connections, and some people's YouTube pages gain celebrity status. YouTube is a popular social media platform for every demographic group; users include people of all ages and are roughly equally divided by gender (Omnicore Agency, 2022).

Instagram

Instagram is another popular social media platform with over 1.4 billion monthly active users (The Small Business Blog, 2022). Instagram is an online photo and video sharing social networking platform and application that is particularly popular among younger generations, with users being roughly equally divided by gender and located around the world (Wikimedia Foundation, 2022a). Instagram allows users to upload media that can be edited with filters and organized by hashtags and geographical tagging, follow trending content, and follow other users and add their content to their own personal feed (Wikimedia Foundation, 2022a). Like Facebook, Instagram posts can include photos or short videos and can be shared publicly or privately with preapproved *followers*. People can communicate with one another directly via *direct message* or by leaving comments and/or reactions (e.g., *liking*) on photos and videos; people can also communicate with each other one-on-one or within a group chat. Instagram is appealing because users can quickly share photos or other visuals with a relatively large group of *followers*. In this way, Instagram helps people to say connected with one another (e.g., family, friends, work colleagues, acquaintances) and with their companion animals, meet new people and groups, and be part of different communities.

TikTok

Currently, TikTok is perhaps the world's most popular social media application among younger generations; it has been described as having "reshaped American culture and hypnotized the world" (Harwell, 2022, para. 5). TikTok offers a variety of short-form (15 seconds to 10 minutes) user videos involving themes such as dance, song, stunts, pranks, and other funny material (Wikimedia Foundation, 2022b); it also offers physical, mental, and spiritual health-related advice by both professionals and nonprofessionals. TikTok has over 1 billion monthly active users and 60% of users are aged between 10 and 29 years (Doyle, 2022). According to a Pew Research Center survey, two-thirds of American teenagers use TikTok and 1 in 6 report that they watch the application almost constantly (Kelly, 2022). TikTok is used mostly for entertainment purposes (watching videos that are created and shared by users) and allows users to follow and be a part of diverse communities. Users can meet new people around the world, in addition to engaging with their already established social networks. Again, people can engage with one another by leaving comments and/or *likes* on videos and can link their social media accounts to their TikTok account for others to access.

Twitter

Twitter is a social media platform that allows users to post and interact with messages known as *tweets*. Registered users can post, like, and retweet tweets with one another, whereas unregistered users can read tweets that are publicly available. Twitter is often used to share breaking news and ideas on current events, trends, research, and resources. Twitter has over 390 million daily active users worldwide and tends to be more popular among men (70.4% of users are male) and young adults or millennials (38.5% of users are aged 25–34 years) (The Social Shepherd, 2022b).

Snapchat

Snapchat is an instant messaging application that is particularly popular among children and youth under the age of 16 years (The Social Shepherd, 2022a). Snapchat has 363 million daily active users worldwide and is most popular among older children and youth (roughly 50% of users are aged between 15 and 25 years; and users are roughly equally divided by gender) (The Social Shepherd, 2022a). Users can quickly share short, one-time messages, pictures, videos, and chronological stories with *friends* (e.g., family, friends, acquaintances), either one-on-one or within a group chat. Snaps can include fun overlays with filters (e.g., 3D world lenses, coloured filters, the current time, local weather, geofilters specific to one's location). Also unique to Snapchat is that messages, pictures, and videos are only available for a short time before they become inaccessible to their recipients. In this way, young people can use creative and fun ways to stay connected with one another.

VSCO

Like Instagram, VSCO is a photo and video editing application that is currently trending and growing in popularity among *Generation Z* users (58.4% of users are aged between 10 and 19 years and 32% of users are aged between 20 and 29 years; and users are roughly equally divided by gender (Dixon, 2022a). VSCO allows users to capture and edit images. Also, users can apply editing tools and preset filters to modify new or existing photos in their camera roll. These photos can then be shared with other social networking services (Wikimedia Foundation, 2022c). Unlike Instagram, VSCO does not offer a privacy option (all posts are public) and fosters social connections and community in a way that is devoid of likes, comments, and follower counts – features that can increase stress among some users.

Overview of Social Media Use and Well-Being

Potential Risks of Social Media Use for Well-Being

Recall in the scenario at the outset of this chapter that Stefan's parents are worried about how some preteens can experience serious bullying and harassment on social media – it turns out that this is a fair concern. Research indicates that social media is sometimes associated with risks to well-being among children, youth, and adults. To begin, there are concerns that increased social media use might negatively impact young people's mental health. Further, some young people show signs of addiction to digital technologies referred to in the DSM-V and ICD-11 as internet gaming disorder. In one study, adolescents who reported an internet gaming disorder or problematic social media use were statistically affected by comorbid clinically relevant depressive symptoms (1 in 3 for adolescents reporting problematic social media use, and 1 in 7 for adolescents reporting an internet gaming disorder; Wartberg et al., 2020). Also, in a scoping review focusing on adolescent social media use and mental health (Vidal et al., 2020), several studies suggested that problematic or addictive social media use may be more common in females and in those starting social media use at a younger age.

Further, concerns also centre on the mental health effects of people's increased use of social media. Findings from one metareview of 34 reviews involving youth and adults (nonclinical samples) suggested an overall (albeit small) negative association between social media use and mental health (Meier & Reinecke, 2020). Specifically, the authors noted that, overall, people who used mobile social media more intensely reported experiencing slightly more internalizing mental health symptoms such as depression, stress, and lower self-esteem (Meier & Reinecke, 2020). In their scoping review, Vidal and colleagues (2020) found that most studies showed a positive and bidirectional association between adolescents' frequency of social media use and adolescent depression and, in some instances, even suicidality. Additionally, research with young people shows a clear link between poorer sleep outcomes (e.g., shorter sleep duration, poor sleep quality) and mobile screen use before going to bed (Robb, 2019), and poor sleeping quality can compromise emotional well-being.

Indeed, as noted by Stefan's parents in the scenario at the outset of this chapter, other risk factors associated with social media use include online bullying or cybervictimization and online exclusion. Conflict or drama may increase adolescents' risk for self-harm and even suicidal behaviour (for reviews, see Naslund et al., 2020; Nesi, 2020). Also, peer influence processes may be heightened online, placing some young people at greater social risk. For instance, there is a concern that people who are exposed to social media content depicting risky behaviours (i.e., alcohol and other substance use, content related to suicide or self-injury) may be more likely to engage in these behaviours themselves. Further, social media might lead people to make unfair or negative social comparisons (e.g., about their physical appearance and abilities), which might heighten risk for depression and body image concerns among young people. Lastly, as noted by Stefan's parents, there is a concern that social media use will replace face-to-face interactions and, in this way, contribute to feelings of loneliness (for reviews, see Naslund et al., 2020; Nesi, 2020).

Potential Benefits of Social Media Use for Well-Being

It turns out that there are also some important well-being benefits associated with the use of social media for children, youth, and adults. Social media platforms offer people a way to connect with a diversity of people at any time of the day and worldwide. People can reach out to family, friends, and other supportive communities in a timely fashion – at the very moment when they are seeking social interactions and/or support. Also, social media platforms might be a more appealing and accessible way for diverse audiences to socially connect (e.g., people who are shy, people using physical mobility aids, people who are sometimes marginalized such as people within BIPOC and 2SLGBTQI+ communities). In this way, social media use can decrease feelings of social isolation and loneliness, facilitate social interactions, foster maintaining daily peer interactions, provide greater access to peer support networks, and foster opportunities for developing new friendships among diverse groups of people and communities. Importantly, social media can create opportunities for equity, diversity, and inclusion in social interactions. In addition to being used for entertainment purposes, social media use can also foster identity exploration and offer opportunities to learn new information and engage in various forms of creative expression.

Additionally, social media platforms and digital mental health tools can offer new opportunities for increasing public awareness about mental health and promote well-being when people access supportive online resources and social networks (Torous et al., 2021). Online social support has been shown to be beneficial to well-being among people experiencing mental health challenges such as depression and anxiety, and the receipt of online social support might also play a protective role for young people who are experiencing mental health challenges such as depression and suicidality (for a review, see Nesi, 2020). A systematic review on the effectiveness of mental health interventions remotely delivered to university students indicates that such approaches have been used for a long time (Davies et al., 2014). Researchers have explored the usefulness of internet-delivered interventions (e.g., mobile-based strategies, use of text and video) to support the social and emotional well-being of university students (Kählke et al., 2019; Klein et al., 2011; Nguyen-Feng et al., 2017; Ruppel & McKinley, 2015). These interventions were not only embedded in programs to promote well-being and prevent the onset of mental health problems but were also used to improve symptoms related to anxiety and depression, among others. Overall, Davies and colleagues (2014) suggest that these programs and interventions may be a valuable resource to promote well-being and offer psychological support to university students. Further, in their scoping review, Vidal and colleagues (2020) noted that some studies have recognized positive effects of social media use on adolescent well-being outcomes including improved depressive symptoms after seeking and receiving social support on Facebook. Another study found that it was possible, over time, for clinically depressed adolescents to successfully shift the way that they used social media from negative (e.g., cyberbullying) to positive (e.g., searching for humorous content) over the course of treatment (Radovic et al., 2016).

To a large extent, research findings support the concerns raised by Stefan's parents in the scenario at the beginning of this chapter about the potential negative impacts of social media use on preteens. At the same time, research findings suggest that Stefan might benefit socially and emotionally by having an Instagram account where he can share pictures of his dog and cat with his friends. Having an Instagram account might help Stefan in making friends and increase his feelings of social connectedness, belonging, and confidence. We now turn to a consideration of how and why people engage in animal-focused social media – how and why do people interact with animals using social media platforms and in what way might this help to enhance learning and support social connections and well-being?

Social Media and Virtual Human-Animal Connections

Animal Pictures, Videos, and Information

It is fair to say that many people use social media to take and share pictures and videos of their beloved companion animals including selfies with animals, animals taking selfies, and animal memes. Still, some people use other digital technologies such as remote pet cameras to continuously monitor their companion animals' health and well-being and sustain their shared emotional connection when they are separated. In terms of animal-focused content, people often use social media platforms (e.g., Facebook, Instagram, TikTok) to share pictures and videos of their companion animals with friends and group members, and social media platforms often have many pages and private groups devoted to animals. They vary in terms of goals and specific topics, and some examples of topics include: (1) groups for owners with animals with disabilities; (2) funny memes and videos about animals; (3) famous animals; (4) rescue and rehoming groups; (5) tips for dog friendly places to visit; (6) groups for professionals working with AAIs; (7) groups about emotional support animals; (8) groups about various breeds of companion animal where "pet lovers" share experiences about their pets; (9) groups about training with tips on how to train your companion animal; and (10) groups focused on wildlife and protection (e.g., Adeyemo, 2019). Also, HAI researchers and practitioners, wildlife conservationists, animal welfarists, and animal rights activists engage social media to share important information about animal research and welfare (e.g., University of British Columbia Okanagan's B.A.R.K.

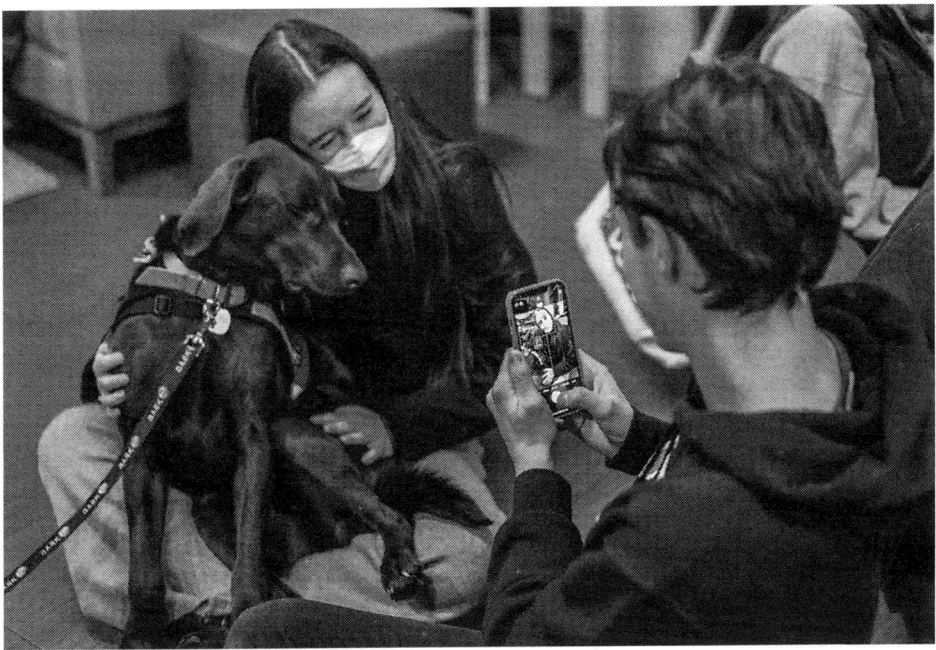

Figure 4.2 A college student using a cell phone to take a picture of another student and therapy dog Skeena

Source: F. L. L. Green Photography

program, University of Saskatchewan's PAWsitive Canine Connections Lab, University of Western Ontario's Dog Cognition Lab).

Social Media Profiles for Animals

In addition to connecting with people they already know and spend time with offline, some people create social media profiles for their animals to meet and connect with new people around their shared passion and love for animals (Golbeck, 2011). Indeed, there is no shortage of social media profiles dedicated to animals, with some profiling only the animals (not their owners) and still others profiling the owner-animal relationship (e.g., *Dogster, Catster, HAM-STERster, Goldfishter, Dogbook* and *Catbook* on Facebook, Golbeck, 2011). These virtual animal profiles are growing in popularity and often include pictures of pets along with their nicknames; birthdays; personality characteristics; favourite toys, foods, and sleeping routines; and other interesting facts.

Famous Pets and Petfluencers

Some people use social media platforms such as Facebook and Instagram to follow interesting and trending animal-focused hashtags (e.g., #animals) which can include themes such as #babyanimal, #cuteanimal, #mammals, #animalkingsdom, #wildlifepictures, and #funpets (e.g., *Best Instagram hashtags for animals*). In this way, some animals have gained celebrity status and have developed a large and loyal social media following (e.g., Boo the Dog, Grumpy Cat, Doug the Pug, Jiff Pom, and Nala Cat). Also, some people engage their

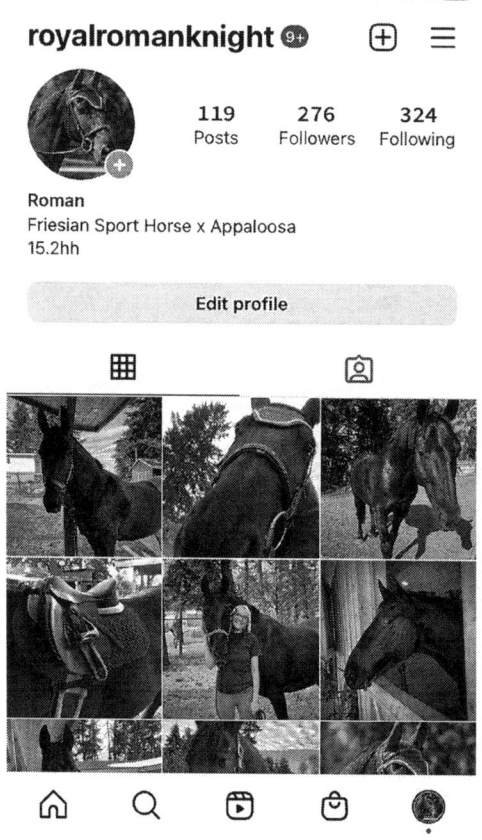

Figure 4.3 Instagram page highlighting a Friesian sport horse named Roman
Source: F. L. L. Green Photography

companion animals to advertise and/or sell products, and these popular animals are known as *Petfluencers* – psychologically, animals are very similar to babies in capturing buyers' attention and interest. One famous *Petfluencer* is Grumpy Cat, an American internet celebrity with an unblinking stare and perpetual "grumpy face." Grumpy Cat gained instant celebrity status in 2012 after her picture was first posted online and went viral. By the time of her death in 2019, Grumpy Cat was an internet sensation and had achieved a following of 2.5 million people on Instagram and millions of views on YouTube. As might be expected, Grumpy Cat's owner formed Grumpy Cat Limited, and Grumpy Cat earned her owner between $1 million and $100 million through merchandising (Andrews, 2021). Today, *Petfluencers* remain a social media phenomenon. In April 2022, the most famous online *Petfluencer* was Jiff Pom, a Pomeranian with 9.8 million Instagram followers, 20.6 million TikTok followers, and 1.3 Facebook followers. Jiff Pom is featured in cute, human-like clothing and has appeared in commercials for companies such as Banana Republic and Target (Dixon, 2022b; Marsh, 2022). In addition to their advertising potential, *Petfluencers* can bring animal lovers together and promote well-being among diverse groups of people around the world (Yarlagadda, 2021; Instagram, n.d.).

Animals in Synchronous, Real-Time Contexts

Some educators and researchers use digital technologies and social media platforms to support humane education initiatives and synchronous, real-time VHAI connections. Also, people can engage with virtual therapy animals in several ways. People can informally seek out relevant online synchronous or asynchronous videos featuring therapy animals. People can also engage with therapy animals in more formal contexts by participating in the online and more structured delivery of well-being support offered within a university or mental health context. Such VHAIs with therapy dogs are increasing in popularity to reduce stress, increase positive affect, and support well-being among psychiatric patients (Scheck et al., 2022), patients receiving palliative care (Kong & Soon, 2022), and university students (Binfet et al., 2022; Dell et al., 2021, Fernandes et al., 2021; Lalonde et al., 2020; Tardif-Williams et al., 2023).

Regarding nontherapy animals, people often individually seek and watch YouTube or TikTok videos of cute animals or engage in digital humane education activities within a classroom or group-based setting. For instance, zoos, aquariums, and animal farms and shelters around the world now feature live animal webcams and interactive cameras offering visitors an immersive virtual experience wherein they can observe animals and explore animal habitats (e.g., take part in a *virtual walk with animals*), thus enabling audiences to diversify how they connect with animals (Thomas, 2020). Using webcams and interactive cameras, people could also observe dogs playing at the park or swimming at the beach and take part in a *virtual walk/play with dog(s) at the* park. Also, these immersive virtual experiences offer human-animal connections characterized by immediacy and intimacy. People can engage in digital animal encounters by accessing live nest, trail, farm, and underwater webcam photos and videos featuring birds, wildlife, farm,

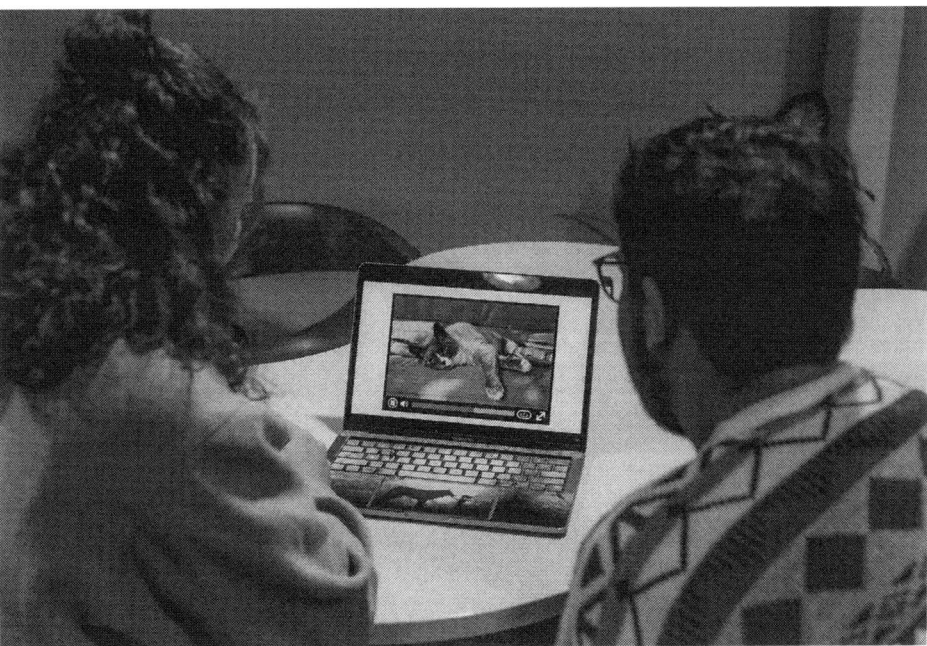

Figure 4.4 Two people sitting at a table watching a video of a cat on a laptop

Source: F. L. L. Green Photography

and fish and marine life. Still other unique and exciting digital encounters with animals include: (1) "creaturely cameos," which involve the livestreaming (on synchronous platforms such as Zoom) of rescued, sanctuary, and farm animals in the United States and United Kingdom; (2) "avatar acquaintances," which involve human-guided virtual visits to the Chernobyl Exclusion Zone organized by an NGO that feeds the dogs living on the site of the 1986 nuclear disaster and (3) "background birding," which involves the use of webcams to continuously livestream the nests of birds of prey – specifically urban peregrine falcons (for a thorough discussion of these digital encounters with animals, see Turnbull et al., 2020).

Why Do People Engage in Social Media That Is Animal-Focused?

Drawing on the available research, we now consider why or what motivates people to engage in social media that is animal-focused and seek out digital encounters with animals. Therefore, we also consider how these virtual human-animal connections might facilitate social connections with both humans and animals and support well-being among social media users.

Enhancing Human-Animal and Social Connections

Bennett and colleagues (2022) examined companion animals' role in improving mental health and reducing stress through the Covid-19 pandemic. The adult participants noted that sharing cat pictures on Facebook helped them to communicate with others. In this way, companion animals were reported to facilitate both in-person and online social interactions by providing topics of conversation to share with others. Charmaraman et al. (2020) found that the more time adolescents (aged 11–16) spent with a dog companion, the more likely they were to browse the internet about animals. Also, the more attached an adolescent was to a dog companion, the more likely an adolescent was to provide and receive online social support. In another study, animal-focused media content helped some students navigate the transition to university (Khalid et al., 2021). Several university students described interacting with their companion animals through video calls, pictures on social media, and videos/pictures of companion animals that they had stored previously or had been sent from home.

In another study, dog owners and cat owners were found to use pet-oriented social networks in different ways. Dog owners reported that they were inclined to use *Dogster* because it allowed them to publicly share pictures and show off their dogs and positive aspects of their shared relationship and obtain helpful advice and information about how to take better care of their dogs (Golbeck, 2011). Dog owners were more likely to create friends for their dogs that were similar in breed and to post more informational messages than cat owners. Using *Dogster* for these reasons likely reflects and enhances positive aspects of the dog-owner bond and relationship. Cat owners tended to use *Catster* to create a broader pool of friends for their cats and to build a stronger sense of virtual community with other users who had cats (Golbeck, 2011). In this way, by sharing a common passion for cats, cat owners have an opportunity to improve online social interactions by building trust and appearing friendlier and more approachable. In a similar study by Golbeck (2009), the previously noted differences in behaviour between dog and cat owners in pet-oriented social networks were extended to divisions between urban and rural users. Specifically, the noted trends between dog and cat owners were more pronounced among people who were living in rural versus urban settings and who were more socially isolated from real-world communities of companion animal owners. It appeared that people were using online pet-oriented social networks to support both social connections and the human-animal bond. Relatedly, pets are sometimes used to promote dating opportunities (e.g., DateMyPet.

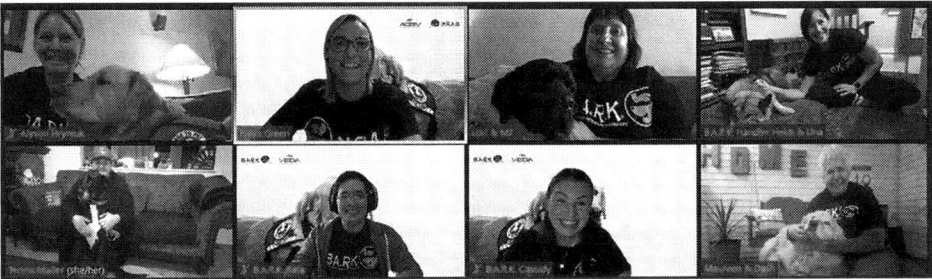

Figure 4.5 A group of handlers from UBC's B.A.R.K. program on a Zoom call with their canine therapeutic partners

Source: F. L. L. Green Photography

com). Future research and practice on VHAIs should consider the different social needs of pet
owners and how VHAIs might equally reflect and enhance aspects of owners' relationships with
their pets.

Anthropomorphizing Animals

Maddox (2020) notes that the cultural practice of engaging in mediated anthropomorphizing on
social media platforms, which involves posting pictures of companion animals along with short
accompanying titles and text, is not new. During the Industrial Revolution, people anthropomorphized their animals by writing letters to each other in their companion animals' voices (Grier,
2006). According to Maddox (2020), creating a companion animal social media account and
curating posts is a self-representational strategy. In posting pictures of our beloved companion
animals on their personalized Instagram accounts, we are not only sharing information about
our pets but also about ourselves. We are curating a "fur baby" self-representation wherein we
reinforce views of ourselves as a loving companion animal parent. Social media offers a digital
space in which to develop and share the "fur baby" identity. Dog blogs or diaries, perhaps, represent a more elaborated version of mediated anthropomorphizing, with dog owners sharing and
reflecting upon their dogs (e.g., activities, emotions, experiences) and their lives with dogs and
do so by using their dogs' voices (Leppänen, 2015).

Examining blogsites of dog owners from around the world, Leppänen (2015) notes that people blog about their dogs for various reasons. First, for many dog owners, blogs function to share
information about their dogs' lives with other dog lovers – they offer a way to socially connect
with other dog owners and share information about dogs' worlds. Still other dog bloggers are
motivated to share and tell stories about their dogs and their life with dogs because they want to
please and entertain other dog enthusiasts. More than this, however, dog blogs reveal information about dog owners, the emotional attachments they share with dogs, and other aspects of the
dog-owner relationship. Leppänen (2015) notes that dog blogging is a form of ventriloquism
that not only highlights dogs' voices but also involves the authentication of the human voice and
humans with particular values and ideologies.

In another study, Austin and Irvine (2020) qualitatively examined how cat owners portrayed
and talked about their cats in an online context via photo sharing with accompanying titles. They
found that cat owners connected with their cats by giving them human (anthropomorphic) characteristics and referred to them as family members that needed to be cared for and sometimes
mourned. Cat owners conceived of their cats as having individuality, thoughts, and emotions.

Like humans, cats were constructed as meaningful *subjects* who fulfilled social and family functions and cat owners used the online space to share anthropomorphized expressions of their cats and their shared bond. Arguably, younger children and adolescents are sharing anthropomorphized representations of animals when they use Snapchat filters to superimpose cute animal face filters onto photos or turn their pets into Disney characters and then share them with their social networks. More intentionally, young people might simply be seeking to recapture an element of their childhood experience.

Animals Are Entertaining and Lucrative

Children and younger adults might be motivated to engage in virtual social media challenges with their companion animals for their entertainment value. Currently, animal-focused TikTok challenges are very popular among young people, and these include the *Call Your Dog Challenge, Triggering Dog Sound Challenge*, and *Mimic Your Cat Challenge*. For the most part, these TikTok challenges are a source of fun and humour and facilitate social connection. Still, as noted previously, other people might be motivated to turn their "fur babies" into media stars or *Petfluencers* to capitalize on animals' marketing and earning potential (e.g., Grumpy Cat).

Supporting Digital Humane Education

Also, as alluded to previously, people might be motivated to engage in digital or immersive encounters with animals via live nest, trail, farm and underwater webcam photos because they are educational and inspiring and offer new ways of perceiving animals as compared with traditional print animal-focused materials. On this note, Cozens-Keeble and colleagues (2021) conducted a study at the Edinburgh Zoo in the UK with children aged 5–15 years who participated in a week-long virtual summer school delivery of zoological education. The study was designed to examine if engagement levels differed for family groups when education was *live, recorded, or activity* based. Study findings showed that overall engagement was higher for the live sessions compared to the recorded content and there was a higher reported nature appreciation at the end of the virtual summer school. The authors conclude by suggesting that the virtual context facilitated social interactions with both humans and animals and engaged and inspired students. In a similar study, Lugosi and Lee (2021) explored the use of virtual reality in the zoo context (at the Royal Zoological Society of Scotland's Edinburgh Zoo) with children aged 13–18 years and adult participants. The younger participants reported that the virtual reality experience allowed them close and personal access to the animals, and the adult participants highlighted the entertainment and potential educational value of the virtual reality experience. Again, we note that educators of diverse students could leverage the potential of virtual reality and immersive experiences as tools to support students' learning and appreciation about animals.

Thus, in addition to including printed animal-focused content, humane educators can offer digital animal encounters and humane education initiatives in the classroom including live nest, trail, farm and underwater webcam photos and videos featuring birds, wildlife, farm, and fish and marine life. In this way, students can learn about a variety of animals and how they behave in their natural habitats and gain viewing access when real-life encounters are not possible. This is important because knowledge about animals and their worlds and a *belief in animal mind,* which involves attributing animals the ability to think, feel, and experience emotions, may influence people's attitudes towards animals as well as their sense of moral duty for animals' welfare (Ellingsen et al., 2010; Hawkins & Williams, 2016; Higgs et al., 2020). Educators can also introduce students to live caterpillar and farm webcams to teach students about biological processes (e.g., caterpillar-to-butterfly metamorphosis, newly born animals with their parents).

Importantly, we submit that new digital technologies and social media offer accessible learning opportunities for diverse children and youth in classrooms around the world, across the socioeconomic spectrum, and regardless of geographical location – educators in diverse contexts (e.g., classrooms, animal shelters, zoos, aquariums) can connect to a broader range of audiences more equitably. Also, researchers and educators could develop specialized curricula in inclusive and sensitive ways to support diverse groups of people including, but not limited to, people who have disabilities and people within BIPOC and 2SLGBTQI+ communities. In this way, VHAIs can be designed to reach diverse audiences and begin to address issues of disparity, diversity, and Indigeneity. Also, it merits noting that these are relatively unobtrusive spaces where animals can be observed and their welfare respected. Thus, educators of diverse students could leverage digital technologies and social media to promote perspective-taking, responsible and compassionate decision-making, and action competence to foster a more humane world.

Seeking to Reduce Anxiety and Stress and Increase Feelings of Awe, Joy, and Calm

Still other people might be motivated to engage in digital or immersive encounters with animals because they reduce feelings of anxiety and stress and elicit a sense of awe and positive emotions such as joy and calm. In one study (Crowley et al., 2021), participants who played a virtual, *immersive ecologies* video game identified a greater number of animal species and reported learning about animal behaviours and interspecies interactions as compared with people who did not play this particular video game. Notably, the study participants highlighted the game's immersive environment as inspiring a range of affective responses including "calm" and "awe." Maddox's (2020) research suggests that people are motivated to post pictures of their companion animals as a way of spreading "joyful" feelings. Social media platforms are all too often replete with negative and discouraging content and the participants' insights suggested that companion animal Instagram accounts may be a way that people work to make their favourite social media platforms more habitable and joyful – rather than being only "cute distractions," animal companion Instagram posts spread joy.

Further, similar to mindfulness practice, quietly observing animals via digital technologies (i.e., watching birds and fish) might help people deal with stress and anxiety by grounding them firmly and restoratively in the present moment. Increasingly, people are listening to animal-themed sounds (e.g., cat purring, horse trotting, cow chewing) via autonomous sensory meridian response (ASMR) videos as a way to experience positive, soothing feelings. Also, virtual connections with animals might provide students with timely *brain breaks* during classroom instruction and help students feel more relaxed and focused on learning. For instance, research by Ein and colleagues (2021, 2022) found that watching prerecorded online videos of dogs (as compared with nature and control videos) decreased subjective anxiety and stress and increased subjective happiness and positive affect among adult participants. In a related study by Ein and colleagues (2020), watching a prerecorded video of a tranquil dog significantly decreased participants' subjective anxiety only, whereas watching a prerecorded video of an active dog significantly decreased participants' subjective stress and anxiety. Further, watching the active dog videos significantly improved subjective alertness and attention when compared with the tranquil dog video – participants also rated the active dog video as more likeable and cuter relative to the tranquil dog video. Also, in another study, watching short YouTube videos of cute baby animals such as kittens and puppies was shown to positively affect veterinary students' mood, their interest in the course, and their self-reported understanding of the course material (Kogan et al., 2018a).

Social media users may seek out videos of cute or funny animals as a form of respite and to create or maintain positive emotions since it appears that online animal videos (and cat videos in particular) can elicit positive emotions. Research by Jacobson et al. (2022) shows that social media animal influencers (or *Petfluencers*) also use affective strategies such as humour and emojis to connect with audiences; this strategy aligns well with audiences as they tend to find online messages with a positive emotional valence to be more engaging (Ki et al., 2020). In a study conducted by Hänninen (2021), people reported that they were motivated to follow *Petfluencers* for five reasons: affection towards pets, entertainment seeking, escaping hard times, curiosity towards pets, and the relationship they form with the pets they follow. When asked why they follow pet animals on Instagram, most of the study respondents described the feel-good factor that the animal content offers them. Still, other innovative research supports the positive impacts to well-being and emotions when people engage with animals in a virtual context. Na and colleagues (2022) explored the potential of mixed reality–based HAIs to reduce stress among university students. Findings showed that the mixed reality–based experiences with virtual cats – where participants could interact using gestures and voice commands – significantly reduced stress (using both self-report and physiological measures) and reduced participants' negative emotions and increased their positive emotions as compared with viewing a slideshow of animal pictures.

Seeking Health and Training Information About Animals

A review of animal-focused content on social media platforms such as Facebook and YouTube suggests that many animal lovers are seeking to share breed-specific personality and behavioural characteristics and animal care and training tips. Also, some people use social media that is animal-focused because they are seeking to share and obtain important health information about their companion animals. Kogan and colleagues (2021) found that Facebook groups are a common source of pet health information among people, with 56.2% of dog owners and 51.8% of cat owners reporting receiving (and sharing) health information through these groups. A similar pattern of findings was found in an online survey with UK pet owners, with 78.6% of respondents reporting that they used the internet as a source of companion animal health information (Kogan et al., 2018b) and in an online survey with Australian pet owners who reported using the internet to obtain pet health information (Kogan et al., 2019). Moving forward, veterinarians could leverage the popular appeal of social media platforms to ensure that people access reliable animal health information and veterinary care. Veterinarians could create a podcast offering information about companion animal health and training and engaging stories such as "A Day in the Life of a Therapy Dog." In addition, people could take part in live virtual veterinary visits with their companion animals. For example, in British Columbia, Canada, veterinarians are offering virtual veterinary care.[1]

Supporting Animal Activism

In her work examining online animal (auto-)biographies, Margo Demello (2018) suggests that online animal biographies may create space for a new way of thinking about animal subjectivity, one that can lead to important changes for the treatment of animals. When people give animals voice on social media and prioritize animal agency, they provide animals a social presence which might contribute to more positive perceptions and treatment of animals. Encouragingly, new research by the American Society for the Prevention of Cruelty to Animals (ASPCA) highlights social media as a helpful tool for animal shelters and rescue organizations in creating new opportunities for fundraising and to increase public awareness and support for animal adoptions (ASPCA, 2018). Also, as noted previously, social media can be used to raise public awareness and support for conservation initiatives and fundraising efforts to support animal adoptions, wildlife, and endangered species. However, social media representations of animals can have damaging effects if people do not know the context of animals' experiences and habitats.

Final Reflections

People seek out digital or social media encounters with animals for a variety of reasons including enhancing human-animal and social connections; anthropomorphizing animals; animals are entertaining and lucrative; reducing anxiety and stress and increasing feelings of awe, joy, and calm; seeking health and training information about animals; and supporting animal activism. It turns out that many of these virtual or social media human-animal encounters help to support people's learning, social connections, and well-being. Turning our attention back to the scenario at the outset of this chapter, research suggests that Stefan might benefit socially and emotionally by having an Instagram account where he can share pictures of his dog and cat with his friends. While there are some risks associated with social media use among young people, having an Instagram account might help Stefan in making friends and increase his feelings of social connectedness, belonging, and confidence. Taken together, the research findings suggest that Stefan's parents might consider a careful and balanced approach in supporting Stefan's request to develop an Instagram account and his use of social media more generally.

When Virtual Human-Animal Interactions Showcase Harm to Animals

Similar to the in-person context, there are animal welfare concerns associated with digital or social media encounters between humans and animals. On the one hand, it might be argued that digital encounters with animals can, to some extent, give voice to animal agency by capturing animals' natural habitats, unpredictability, and aliveness in a way that is largely free from human mediation (for a discussion, see von Essen et al., 2021). "On the other hand, von Essen et al. (2021) note that such virtual intimacy is asymmetrical and problematic insomuch as it enters animals into relations of care and commodification (i.e., "Disneyfication" of animals where animals are anthropomorphized, rendering them akin to cartoon-like characters; editing behaviours to their most visually interesting forms"). Here, we would be remiss if we did not raise awareness about animal welfare within virtual or social media contexts.

Social media platforms themselves cannot always do enough to prevent and monitor posts that violate regulations and national laws safeguarding animals from cruelty and illegal activities. Unfortunately, it is the case that social media sometimes features a range of intentional acts of animal abuse and cruelty. Sometimes people unintentionally engage in acts that are harmful to animals. As one example, animal advocates warn that the seemingly harmless and fun TikTok *Hole Digging Challenge* can create a deadly hazard for sea turtles (Andrews, 2022). Also, YouTube videos of endangered and exotic species and animals that should not be kept as companion animals are sometimes cited as the impetus for people to pursue keeping those animals as pets (Nekaris et al., 2013). The slow loris is an example of an animal that is further endangered for being cute due to a video that was first uploaded on social media in 2009 and quickly went viral. The video features Sonya, an overweight slow loris, who is being kept as a companion animal and is being "tickled." Unfortunately, such videos on social media can perpetuate misperceptions of animal welfare, thwart animal conservation efforts, and drive people's desire for keeping endangered and exotic animals as pets, compromising animal welfare (Nekaris et al., 2013).

Social media contexts can also moderate perceptions of animals. Riddle and MacKay (2020) presented adults participants with mock-up pages from a social media site (i.e., Facebook page created by the researchers) showing a primate. Half the participants were shown a negative story and the other half were shown a positive story. When participants were presented with the anti-exotic pet narrative, they perceived the primate to be more stressed – suggesting that social media sites may moderate attitudes to animal welfare issues. Lenzi et al. (2020) also note that social media or digital encounters with animals in the form of "viral" videos and "wildlife selfies" can influence public perceptions of wild animals and compromise their welfare. Digital or immersive encounters often present wild animals as ideal companion animals. These inappropriate depictions of wild animals as tame or humanized can make it increasingly desirable to keep them as companion animals and drive the illegal wildlife trade and promote harmful tourism encounters with wild animals. Vander Meer (2022) warns that the "collector's gaze" or practice of getting up close to take "wildlife selfies" has led to the death of other animals and places people in dangerous situations as they strive to capture unique images (e.g., tourists taking selfies with bison in Yellowstone National Park). Also, social media can also be used to actively encourage misrepresentations of animal worlds. For instance, Linné (2016) analyzed two examples (one Instagram and one Facebook) of the Swedish dairy industry, and they argued that the Swedish dairy industry's social media presence often misrepresented the cows as willingly producing milk for a caring and compassionate industry.

Conclusion

Human-animal interactions within virtual and social media contexts are growing in popularity and rapidly changing. In this chapter, we discussed the increasingly important role of social media in people's lives, outlined several platforms currently popular with both younger people and older generations, and raised some of the benefits and risks associated with social media use. We then considered the many ways that animals tend to feature prevalently within virtual and social media contexts ranging from sharing pictures and videos of cute animals on social media to engaging with therapy animals and enjoying virtual visits to zoos, aquariums, animal sanctuaries, and wildlife centres. We then considered why people seek animal-focused digital and social media experiences and, in doing so, outlined some of the potential risks and social and well-being benefits for users. We concluded with a discussion of animal welfare concerns that arise via virtual human-animal encounters. In the next chapter, we turn to a consideration of ways to safeguard animal welfare within virtual and social media contexts. We hope that researchers, educators, and practitioners alike will consider how they might leverage social media and virtual interactions between animals and diverse people to support learning, social connections, and well-being.

Note

1   www.kelownanow.com/watercooler/news/news/Provincial/Cats_and_dogs_in_BC_SPCA_animal_shelters_to_benefit_from_virtual_vet_care/

References

Adeyemo, H. (2019). The 14 best wildlife Instagram accounts to follow. *Signature Safaris*. Retrieved October 17, 2022, from www.signatureafricansafaris.com/best-wildlife-instagram-accounts/

Ahmed, Y. A., Ahmad, M. N., Ahmad, N., & Zakaria, N. H. (2019). Social media for knowledge-sharing: A systematic literature review. *Telematics and Informatics*, *37*, 72–112. https://doi.org/10.1016/j.tele.2018.01.015

Andrews, B. (2022). Hole digging TikTok Challenge creates deadly hazard for sea turtles, wildlife advocates warn. *WJXT*. Retrieved October 21, 2022, from www.news4jax.com/news/local/2022/07/16/hole-digging-tiktok-challenge-creates-deadly-hazard-for-sea-turtles-wildlife-advocates-warn/

Andrews, T. M. (2021). Grumpy cat owner awarded over $700,000 in lawsuit. cat still won't smile. *The Washington Post*. Retrieved October 17, 2022, from www.washingtonpost.com/news/morning-mix/wp/2018/01/24/grumpy-cat-owners-awarded-over-700000-in-lawsuit-cat-still-wont-smile/

ASPCA. (2018). *New research points to social media as important tool for animal shelters and rescues*. Retrieved October 21, 2022, from www.aspca.org/about-us/press-releases/new-research-points-social-media-important-tool-animal-shelters-and-rescues.

Austin, J., & Irvine, L. (2020). "A very photogenic cat": Personhood, social status, and online cat photo sharing. *Anthrozoös, 33*(3), 441–450. https://doi.org/10.1080/08927936.2020.1746533

Barnhart, B. (2022). 20 must-know Facebook stats for marketers in 2022. *Sprout Social*. Retrieved October 17, 2022, from https://sproutsocial.com/insights/facebook-stats-for-marketers/?amp

Bennett, B., Cosh, S., Thepsourinthone, J., & Lykins, A. (2022). A mixed-methods assessment of human well-being related to the presence of companion animals during the COVID-19 pandemic. *People and Animals: The International Journal of Research and Practice, 5*(1). https://docs.lib.purdue.edu/paij/vol5/iss1/5

Binfet, J. T., Tardif-Williams, C., Draper, Z. A., Green, F. L. L., Singal, A., Rousseau, C. X., & Roma, R. (2022). Virtual canine comfort: A randomized controlled trial of the effects of a canine-assisted intervention supporting undergraduate wellbeing. *Anthrozoös, 35*(6), 809–832. https://doi.org/10.1080/08927936.2022.2062866

Charmaraman, L., Mueller, M. K., & Richer, A. M. (2020). The role of pet companionship in online and offline social interactions in adolescence. *Child and Adolescent Social Work Journal, 37*(6), 589–599. https://doi.org/10.1007/s10560-020-00707-y

Cozens-Keeble, E. H., Arnold, R., Newman, A., & Freeman, M. S. (2021). It's virtually summer, can the zoo come to you? Zoo summer school engagement in an online setting. *Journal of Zoological and Botanical Gardens, 2*(45), 625–635. https://doi.org/10.3390/jzbg2040045

Crowley, E. J., Silk, M. J., & Crowley, S. L. (2021). The educational value of virtual ecologies in Red Dead Redemption 2. *People and Nature, 3*(6), 1229–1243. https://doi.org/10.1002/pan3.10242

Davies, E. B., Morriss, R., & Glazebrook, C. (2014). Computer-delivered and web-based interventions to improve depression, anxiety, and psychological well-being of university students: A systematic review and meta-analysis. *Journal of Medical Internet Research, 16*(5). https://doi.org/10.2196/jmir.3142

Dell, C., Williamson, L., McKenzie, H., Carey, B., Cruz, M., Gibson, M., & Pavelich, A. (2021). A commentary about lessons learned: Transitioning a therapy dog program online during the COVID-19 pandemic. *Animals, 11*(3), 914. https://doi.org/10.3390/ani11030914

DeMello, M. (2018). Online animal (auto-)biographies: What does it mean when we "give animals a voice?". In A. Krebber & M. Roscher (Eds.), *Animal Biography. Palgrave Studies in Animals and Literature*. Palgrave Macmillan. https://doi.org/10.1007/978-3-319-98288-5_13

Dixon, S. (2022a). U.S. VSCO Mau users by age 2021. *Statista*. Retrieved October 17, 2022, from www.statista.com/statistics/1125147/vsco-us-users-age/

Dixon, S. (2022b). Instagram: Most-followed Petfluencers worldwide 2020. *Statista*. Retrieved October 17, 2022, from www.statista.com/statistics/785972/most-followers-instagram-petfluencers/

Doyle, B. (2022). TikTok statistics – everything you need to know. *Wallaroo Media*. Retrieved October 17, 2022, from https://wallaroomedia.com/blog/social-media/tiktok-statistics/

Ein, N., Gervasio, J., Reed, M. J., & Vickers, K. (2022). Effects on wellbeing of exposure to dog videos before a stressor. *Anthrozoös*, 1–19. https://doi.org/10.1080/08927936.2022.2149925

Ein, N., Reed, M. J., & Vickers, K. (2020). Effect of tranquil and active video representations of an unfamiliar dog on subjective mental states. *Society & Animals, 30*(4), 445–460. https://doi.org/10.1163/15685306-bja10019

Ein, N., Reed, M. J., & Vickers, K. (2021). The effect of dog videos on subjective and physiological responses to stress. *Anthrozoös, 35*(3), 463–482. https://doi.org/10.1080/08927936.2021.1999606

Ellingsen, K., Zanella, A. J., Bjerkås, E., & Indrebø, A. (2010). The relationship between empathy, perception of pain and attitudes toward pets among Norwegian dog owners. *Anthrozoös*, *23*(3), 231–243. https://doi.org/10.2752/175303710x12750451258931

Fernandes, A., Chae, Y. S., & South, C. S. (2021). An exploratory analysis of virtual delivery alternatives for university-based animal assisted activities during COVID-19. *Purdue e-Pubs*. Retrieved October 19, 2022, from https://docs.lib.purdue.edu/paij/vol4/iss1/6

Golbeck, J. (2009). On the internet, everybody knows you're A dog: The human-pet relationship in online social networks. *CHI'09 Extended Abstracts on Human Factors in Computing Systems*, April, 4495–5000. https://doi.org/10.1145/1520340.1520689

Golbeck, J. (2011). The more people I meet, the more I like my dog: A study of pet-oriented social networks on the web. *First Monday*, *16*, 2–7. https://doi.org/10.5210/fm.v16i2.2859

Grier, K. (2006). *Pets in America: A history*. Harvest Books.

Hannahcurrey. (2022). Digital 2022: Another year of bumper growth. *We Are Social UK*. Retrieved October 17, 2022, from https://wearesocial.com/uk/blog/2022/01/digital-2022-another-year-of-bumper-growth-2/

Hänninen, C. (2021). *Why does my neighbor's labradoodle have eight million followers on . . .* Retrieved October 19, 2022, from https://helda.helsinki.fi/dhanken/bitstream/handle/10227/441217/H%C3%A4nninen_Carina.pdf

Harwell, D. (2022). How TikTok ate the internet. *The Washington Post*. Retrieved October 17, 2022, from www.washingtonpost.com/technology/interactive/2022/tiktok-popularity/

Hawkins, R. D., & Williams, J. M. (2016). Children's beliefs about animal minds (child-BAM): Associations with positive and negative child – animal interactions. *Anthrozoös*, *29*(3), 503–519. https://doi.org/10.1080/08927936.2016.1189749

Higgs, M. J., Bipin, S., & Cassaday, H. J. (2020). Man's best friends: Attitudes towards the use of different kinds of animal depend on belief in different species' mental capacities and purpose of use. *Royal Society Open Science*, *7*(2), 191162. https://doi.org/10.1098/rsos.191162

Instagram. (n.d.). *Animals lover on Instagram*. Retrieved October 17, 2022, from www.instagram.com/reel/Cbjf6AQFznh/?igshid=MDJmNzVkMjY

Jacobson, J., Hodson, J., & Mittelman, R. (2022). PUP-ularity contest: The advertising practices of popular animal influencers on Instagram. *Technological Forecasting and Social Change*, *174*, 121226. https://doi.org/10.1016/j.techfore.2021.121226

Kählke, F., Berger, T., Schulz, A., Baumeister, H., Berking, M., Cuijpers, P., Bruffaerts, R., Auerbach, R. P., Kessler, R. C., & Ebert, D. D. (2019). Efficacy and cost-effectiveness of an unguided, internet-based self-help intervention for Social Anxiety Disorder in university students: Protocol of a randomized controlled trial. *BMC Psychiatry*, *19*(1). https://doi.org/10.1186/s12888-019-2125-4

Kelly, H. (2022). Teens have fled Facebook but are loyal to YouTube, poll shows. *The Washington Post*. Retrieved October 17, 2022, from www.washingtonpost.com/technology/2022/08/10/teens-social-pew/

Khalid, A., Rogers, A., Vicary, E., & Brooks, H. (2021). Human-animal interaction to support well-being at university: Experiences of undergraduate students in the UK. *People and Animals: The International Journal of Research and Practice*, *4*(2). https://docs.lib.purdue.edu/paij/vol4/iss1/2/

Ki, C.-W. C., Cuevas, L. M., Chong, S. M., & Lim, H. (2020). Influencer marketing: Social media influencers as human brands attaching to followers and yielding positive marketing results by fulfilling needs. *Journal of Retailing and Consumer Services*, *55*, 102133. https://doi.org/10.1016/j.jretconser.2020.102133

Klein, B., Meyer, D., Austin, D. W., & Kyrios, M. (2011). Anxiety online – a virtual clinic: Preliminary outcomes following completion of five fully automated treatment programs for anxiety disorders and symptoms. *Journal of Medical Internet Research*, *13*(4). https://doi.org/10.2196/jmir.1918

Kogan, L. R., Hazel, S. J., & Oxley, J. A. (2019). A pilot study of Australian pet owners who engage in social media and their use, experience and views of online pet health information. *Australian Veterinary Journal*, *97*(11), 433–439. https://doi.org/10.1111/avj.12870

Kogan, L. R., Hellyer, P. W., Clapp, T. R., Suchman, E., McLean, J., & Schoenfeld-Tacher, R. (2018a). Use of short animal-themed videos to enhance veterinary students' mood, attention, and understanding of pharmacology lectures. *Journal of Veterinary Medical Education*, *45*(2), 188–194. https://doi.org/10.3138/jvme.1016-162r

Kogan, L. R., Little, S., & Oxley, J. (2021). Dog and cat owners' use of online Facebook groups for pet health information. *Health Information & Libraries Journal*, *38*(3), 203–223. https://doi.org/10.1111/hir.12351

Kogan, L. R., Oxley, J. A., Hellyer, P., Schoenfeld, R., & Rishniw, M. (2018b). UK pet owners' use of the internet for online pet health information. *Veterinary Record*, *182*(21), 601. https://doi.org/10.1136/vr.104716

Kong, C., & Soon, S. M. (2022). Virtual volunteering during the COVID-19 pandemic: Case studies of virtual animal-assisted activities in a Singapore hospice. *Journal of Social Work in End-of-Life & Palliative Care*, *18*(3), 203–215. https://doi.org/10.1080/15524256.2022.2105472

Lalonde, R., Dell, C., & Claypool, T. (2020). Paws your stress: The student experience of therapy dog programming. *Canadian Journal for New Scholars in Education/Revue canadienne des jeunes chercheures et chercheurs en éducation*. Retrieved October 19, 2022, from https://journalhosting.ucalgary.ca/index.php/cjnse/article/view/69530

Lenzi, C., Speiran, S., & Grasso, C. (2020). "Let me take a selfie": Implications of social media for public perceptions of wild animals. *Society & Animals*, *31*(1), 64–83. https://doi.org/10.1163/15685306-bja10023

Leppänen, S. (2015). Dog blogs as ventriloquism: Authentication of the human voice. *Discourse, Context & Media*, *8*, 63–73. https://doi.org/10.1016/j.dcm.2015.05.005

Linné, T. (2016). Cows on Facebook and Instagram. *Television & New Media*, *17*(8), 719–733. https://doi.org/10.1177/1527476416653811

Lugosi, Z., & Lee, P. C. (2021). A case study exploring the use of virtual reality in the zoo context. *Animal Behavior and Cognition*, *8*(4), 576–588. https://doi.org/10.26451/abc.08.04.09.2021

Maddox, J. (2020). The secret life of pet Instagram accounts: Joy, resistance, and commodification in the internet's cute economy. *New Media & Society*, *23*(11), 3332–3348. https://doi.org/10.1177/1461444820956345

Marsh, E. (2022). National pet day: The top pet influencers + insights. *StatSocial*. Retrieved October 17, 2022, from www.statsocial.com/national-pet-day-insights-and-influencers

Meese, J. (2014). "It belongs to the internet": Animal images, attribution norms and the politics of Amateur Media Production. *M/C Journal*, *17*(2). https://doi.org/10.5204/mcj.782

Meier, A., & Reinecke, L. (2020). Computer-mediated communication, social media, and mental health: A conceptual and empirical meta-review. *Communication Research*, *48*(8), 1182–1209. https://doi.org/10.1177/0093650220958224

Na, H., Park, S., & Dong, S.-Y. (2022). Mixed reality-based interaction between human and virtual cat for Mental Stress Management. *Sensors*, *22*(3), 1159. https://doi.org/10.3390/s22031159

Naslund, J. A., Bondre, A., Torous, J., & Aschbrenner, K. A. (2020). Social media and mental health: Benefits, risks, and opportunities for research and Practice. *Journal of Technology in Behavioral Science*, *5*(3), 245–257. https://doi.org/10.1007/s41347-020-00134-x

Nekaris, K. A. I., Campbell, N., Coggins, T. G., Rode, E. J., & Nijman, V. (2013). Correction: tickled to death: Analysing public perceptions of 'cute' videos of threatened species (slow lorises – *Nycticebus* spp.) on web 2.0 sites. *PLoS One*, *8*(8). https://doi.org/10.1371/annotation/7afd7924-ca2b-4b9c-ac1b-2cc656b3bf42

Nesi, J. (2020). The impact of social media on youth mental health. *North Carolina Medical Journal*, *81*(2), 116–121. https://doi.org/10.18043/ncm.81.2.116

Nguyen-Feng, V. N., Greer, C. S., & Frazier, P. (2017). Using online interventions to deliver college student mental health resources: Evidence from randomized clinical trials. *Psychological Services*, *14*(4), 481–489. https://doi.org/10.1037/ser0000154

Omnicore Agency. (2022, August 2002). 63 *Facebook statistics you need to know in 2022 – Omnicore*. Retrieved October 17, 2022, from www.omnicoreagency.com/facebook-statistics/

Radovic, A., Gmelin, T., Stein, B. D., & Miller, E. (2016). Depressed adolescents' positive and negative use of social media. *Journal of Adolescence*, *55*(1), 5–15. https://doi.org/10.1016/j.adolescence.2016.12.002

Rault, J.-L. (2015). Pets in the digital age. Live, robot, or virtual? *Frontiers in Veterinary Science*, *2*(11), https://doi.org/10.3389/fvets.2015.00011

Riddle, E., & MacKay, J. R. (2020). Social media contexts moderate perceptions of animals. *Animals*, *10*(5), 845. https://doi.org/10.3390/ani10050845

Robb, E. (2019). The new normal: Parents, teens, screens, and sleep in the United States. *Common Sense Media*. Retrieved October 17, 2022, from www.commonsensemedia.org/videos/the-new-normal-parents-teens-screens-and-sleep-in-the-united-states

Ruppel, E. K., & McKinley, C. J. (2015). Social support and social anxiety in use and perceptions of online mental health resources: Exploring social compensation and enhancement. *Cyberpsychology, Behavior, and Social Networking, 18*(8), 462–467. https://doi.org/10.1089/cyber.2014.0652

Scheck, H., Williamson, L., & Dell, C. A. (2022). Understanding psychiatric patients' experience of virtual animal-assisted therapy sessions during the COVID-19 pandemic. *Purdue e-Pubs*. Retrieved October 18, 2022, from https://docs.lib.purdue.edu/paij/vol5/iss1/6

Tardif-Williams, C. Y., Binfet, J. T., Green, F. L. L., Roma, R., Akshat, S., Rousseau, C. X., & Godard, R. J. (2023). When therapy dogs provide virtual comfort: Exploring university students' insights and perspectives. *People and Animals: The International Journal of Research and Practice, 6*(1), 1–17. https://docs.lib.purdue.edu/paij/vol6/iss1/5

The Small Business Blog. (2022). *How many people use Instagram in 2022? (Instagram statistics)*. Retrieved October 17, 2022, from https://thesmallbusinessblog.net/instagram-statistics/

The Social Shepherd. (2022a). *21 essential Snapchat statistics you need to know in 2022*. Retrieved October 17, 2022, from https://thesocialshepherd.com/blog/snapchat-statistics

The Social Shepherd. (2022b). *22 essential Twitter statistics you need to know in 2022*. Retrieved October 17, 2022, from https://thesocialshepherd.com/blog/twitter-statistics

Thomas, S. (2020). Social change for conservation – the world zoo and aquarium conservation education strategy. *International Zoo Educators Association*. Retrieved October 19, 2022, from https://izea.net/the-waza-education-strategy/

Torous, J., Bucci, S., Bell, I. H., Kessing, L. V., Faurholt-Jepsen, M., Whelan, P., Carvalho, A. F., Keshavan, M., Linardon, J., & Firth, J. (2021). The growing field of digital psychiatry: Current evidence and the future of apps, social media, chatbots, and virtual reality. *World Psychiatry, 20*(3), 318–335. https://doi.org/10.1002/wps.20883

Turnbull, J., Searle, A., & Adams, W. M. (2020). Quarantine encounters with digital animals: More-than-human geographies of Lockdown Life. *Journal of Environmental Media, 1*(1), 6.1–6.10. https://doi.org/10.1386/jem_00027_1

Vander Meer, E. (2022). Creating distance or proximity?: How wild lives are told through remote camera viewing. *Multispecies Storytelling in Intermedial Practices*, 279–302. https://doi.org/10.53288/0338.1.17

Vidal, C., Lhaksampa, T., Miller, L., & Platt, R. (2020). Social media use and depression in adolescents: A scoping review. *International Review of Psychiatry, 32*(3), 235–253. https://doi.org/10.1080/09540261.2020.1720623

Vogels, E. A., Gelles-Watnick, R., & Massarat, N. (2022). Teens, social media and technology 2022. *Pew Research Center: Internet, Science & Tech*. Retrieved October 17, 2022, from www.pewresearch.org/internet/2022/08/10/teens-social-media-and-technology-2022/

von Essen, E., Turnbull, J., Searle, A., Jørgensen, F. A., Hofmeester, T. R., & van der Wal, R. (2021). Wildlife in the digital Anthropocene: Examining human-animal relations through surveillance technologies. *Environment and Planning E: Nature and Space, 6*(1), 679–699. https://doi.org/10.1177/25148486211061704

Wartberg, L., Kriston, L., & Thomasius, R. (2020). Internet gaming disorder and problematic social media use in a representative sample of German adolescents: Prevalence estimates, comorbid depressive symptoms and related psychosocial aspects. *Computers in Human Behavior, 103*, 31–36. https://doi.org/10.1016/j.chb.2019.09.014

Wikimedia Foundation. (2022a). Instagram. *Wikipedia*. Retrieved October 17, 2022, from https://en.wikipedia.org/wiki/Instagram

Wikimedia Foundation. (2022b). TikTok. *Wikipedia*. Retrieved October 17, 2022, from https://en.wikipedia.org/wiki/TikTok

Wikimedia Foundation. (2022c). VSCO. *Wikipedia*. Retrieved October 17, 2022, from https://en.wikipedia.org/wiki/VSCO

Yarlagadda, T. (2021). Instagram dogs and TikTok cats are saving animals – and the environment. *Inverse*. Retrieved October 17, 2022, from www.inverse.com/science/how-petfluencers-can-be-a-force-for-good/amp

5 Safeguarding Animal Welfare in a Virtual Context

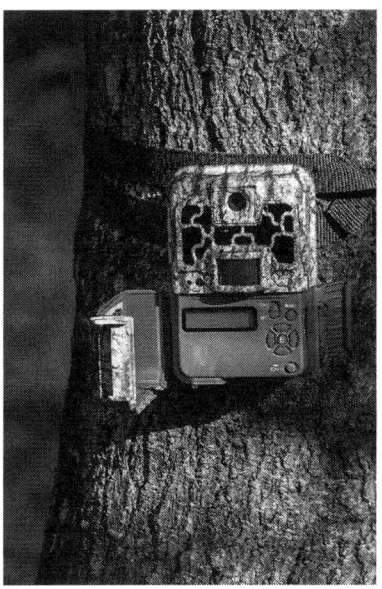

Figure 5.1 Wildlife trail cam
Source: Pixabay

Scenario

Trail cams, fast food, and urban wildlife

Imagine a popular vlogger rigging up a trail camera to capture images of wildlife in the heart of downtown Vancouver's famous urban forest, Stanley Park. To the surprise of the vlogger and viewers, images of a wide variety of wildlife are captured and reveal the trail to be well-used by animals navigating their way through the city, presumably as they seek to avoid contact with humans. Popularity of the trail cam grows, and individual animals using the trail develop fan bases comprised of devoted and loyal viewers. A bridge in the background reveals the location of the trail which subsequently draws the heightened attention of viewers and enthusiasts keen to see wildlife up close to complement their virtual viewing experiences. Some viewers begin posting comments suggesting that leaving food to attract animals within the viewing frame of the camera could enhance the public's chances of seeing more animals

DOI: 10.4324/9781003327868-5

whilst encouraging the animals to spend more time in front of the camera. Fast food contain-ers are soon seen in the trail cam frame to attract wildlife. It is here we see the intersection of technology and animal welfare clash.

Questions for Reflection

1. What considerations for animal welfare arise within virtual contexts?
2. How is animal welfare safeguarded for wildlife living in public spaces?
3. Whose responsibility is it to safeguard the welfare of wildlife?

> Interests in the welfare of animals and how animals should be treated are influenced by a complex set of personal motivations, and different stakeholders will evaluate welfare through different frames of references, often subjectively.
>
> (McBride & Baugh, 2022, p. 129)

Our opening scenario was inspired by a popular vlogger's stunt in which a pizza was left in a forest in front of a trail cam. Titled "What happens to a pizza left in the woods" (Ace Vlogs, 2023), this video has, at the time of print, over 2 million views and illustrates the complexities surrounding technology, social media, wildlife, and animal welfare. Certainly, in cases such as this where viewership contributes to monetary gains for the individuals who create digital content, we can, oftentimes, see concerns for animal welfare take a backseat. Within a virtual context, we would categorize the leaving of a pizza in the forest as meeting, albeit in a misguided and manipulated way, the curiosity of the public to gain access to, or virtually interact with, animals. It is not only in ungoverned spaces such as this where a trail camera is used to capture animal reactions to a pizza left in the woods that issues of animal welfare arise. We also see welfare issues emerge front and centre when domestic animals participate in structured in-person interactions with humans.

Admittedly, concerns and protocols to safeguard the welfare of animals participating in animal-assisted interventions (AAIs) have struggled to keep up with the burgeoning field of HAIs. That is, implementation of AAIs has forged forward to see programs introduced within and across a variety of settings serving a variety of populations and the careful consideration of animal welfare can, oftentimes, be left lagging (Howe et al., 2022). Considerations of ani-mal welfare within AAIs remains a nascent area of discussion, implementation, and study, and the aims of this chapter are to define animal welfare, examine it within a virtual context, and elucidate considerations surrounding the optimal safeguarding of animal welfare within the context of virtual human-animal interactions. In this chapter, we draw on emerging research and scholarship on animal welfare within the context of HAIs and AAIs and consider animal welfare within a virtual context.

As dogs are most frequently involved with AAIs (Glenk & Foltin, 2021; Ng et al., 2019; Wagner et al., 2022), much of the research on therapy animal welfare focuses on dogs' well-being. In a recent systematic review of studies conducted between 1987 and 2022, Wagner and colleagues (2022) identified that the majority of AAI-themed publications situated dogs as therapeutic partners at twice the rate of horses, followed by infrequent mention of cats, guinea pigs, and farm animals. We recognize this imbalance in the animals participating in studies and have done our best to take a broad lens on animal welfare spanning a range of species from therapy dogs to horses to wildlife. As illustrations of animal welfare considera-tions beyond therapy dogs, readers are encouraged to consult the work of Muvhali (2018), whose graduate research examined ostrich welfare in HAIs; the work of Frye (2021) and De

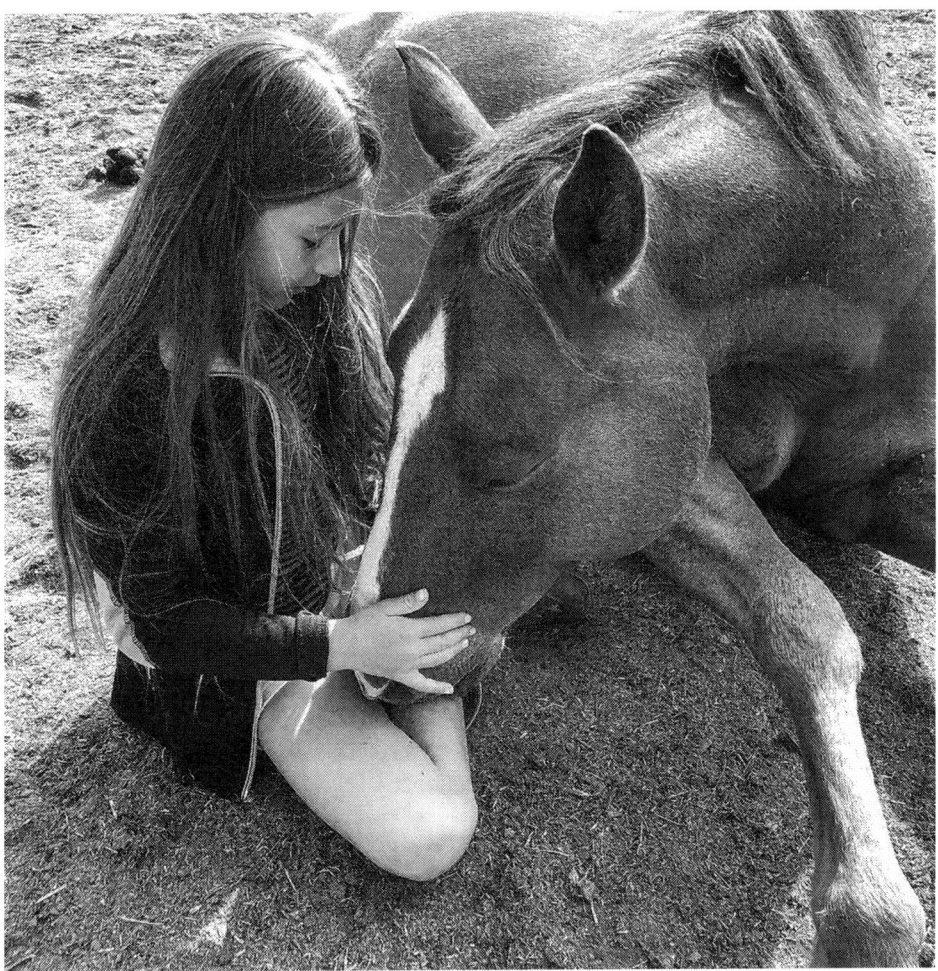

Figure 5.2 A child shares a tender moment with her horse Donnie

Source: Krista Evans Photography

Santis et al. (2017), who advocate for equine welfare in horses working in therapeutic and educational contexts; and the work of Gut and colleagues (2018), who assessed the impact of HAI on guinea pigs.

Defining Animal Welfare Within the Context of Animal-Assisted Interventions

> Not all human-animal interactions are successful for either party or for the animal alone.
>
> (McBride & Baugh, 2022, p. 134)

Within a broad context, animal welfare is often measured in comparison to the benchmark of "The Five Freedoms" (Webster, 1994). Originally proffered to promote welfare considerations in livestock, the Five Freedoms are comprised of freedom: (1) from hunger, thirst, and malnutrition; (2) from discomfort; (3) from pain, injury, or disease; (4) from fear and distress; and (5) of behavioural expression. We see these Five Freedoms referenced in contemporary writing on animal welfare in AAI (e.g., Barker & Gee, 2021; McBride & Baugh, 2022; Mellor, 2017; Ng et al., 2015), and although they provide a benchmark or guidelines for animals working broadly within HAI, a more nuanced examination of welfare is required for animals working more specifically in AAIs (see Barker & Gee, 2021 and McBride & Baugh, 2022 for discussions of the limitations of the Five Freedoms vis-à-vis HAI). Extending the Five Freedoms model is the collective work of Barker and Gee (2021), McBride and Baugh (2022), Nussbaum and Sen (2004), and Ng and colleagues (2015), who, among others, argue that we must move beyond a needs or care perspective evident in the Five Freedoms model. Rather, welfare should address the animal's *affective* experience and be viewed as a reflection of both compassionate relationships and the animal's potential to flourish.

As a reflection of compassionate relationships within AAIs, Glenk and Foltin (2021, p. 227) argue, "The practice of animals merely tolerating the interaction and following the handler's commands is explicitly criticized (IAHAIO, 2018; Pet Partners, 2018)." HAI researchers have advocated for "low stress handling techniques" and "fear free principles" to guide interactions between animals and humans (Binfet & Hartwig, 2020; Overall, 2013; Scalia et al., 2017; Yin, 2009). Animals are not to be coerced or manipulated by handlers to interact with humans in order for humans to derive well-being benefits at the animal's expense. In a recent position paper by Horrowitz (2021) titled "Considering the 'dog' in dog-human interaction," Horrowitz acknowledges the utilitarian approach many have taken with respect to working with animals in AAIs: "In HAI research, the animal is a quiet partner, useful only for the effect their presence has on the person, and rarely considered in and of themselves" (p. 1). Rather, the animal's well-being must be considered as integral to the interaction and, increasingly, researchers are heeding the call to understand the animal's affective experience within AAI sessions (see Hatch, 2007; Sarrafchi et al., 2022; Silas et al., 2019 for examples).

Defining animal welfare within the context of virtual HAIs is important as the needs of therapy animals are unique and distinct to the contexts in which they work and the clients they strive to support. Leaning on the early work of Broom (1986), we see animal welfare defined as "the state of an animal as regards its attempts to cope with its environment" (p. 524). In the following definition proffered by Ng and colleagues (2015, p. 359), we again see emphasis on animals adapting to their environment:

> Very good welfare and well-being status is characterized as a state in which an animal is free from distress most of the time, is in good physical health, exhibits a substantial range of species-typical behaviors, and is able to cope effectively with environmental stimuli (Hetts et al., 1992; Novak & Drewsen, 1989).

Undergirding this ability to cope with the environment is the animal's consent to engage in activities organized within these environments. The role of consent is garnering increased attention from researchers, especially within the context of research exploring the effects of therapy dogs on human well-being (see Glenk, 2017). Returning to the work of Horrowitz (2021) referenced previously, the role of consent is articulated within the broader context of AAI:

> I recommend that researchers and handlers be mindful of the animal's perspectives of the activities they are engaging in; strive not just for lack of poor welfare but also the presence of positive welfare; and work towards standards of affirmative consent.
>
> (Horrowitz, 2021, p. 5)

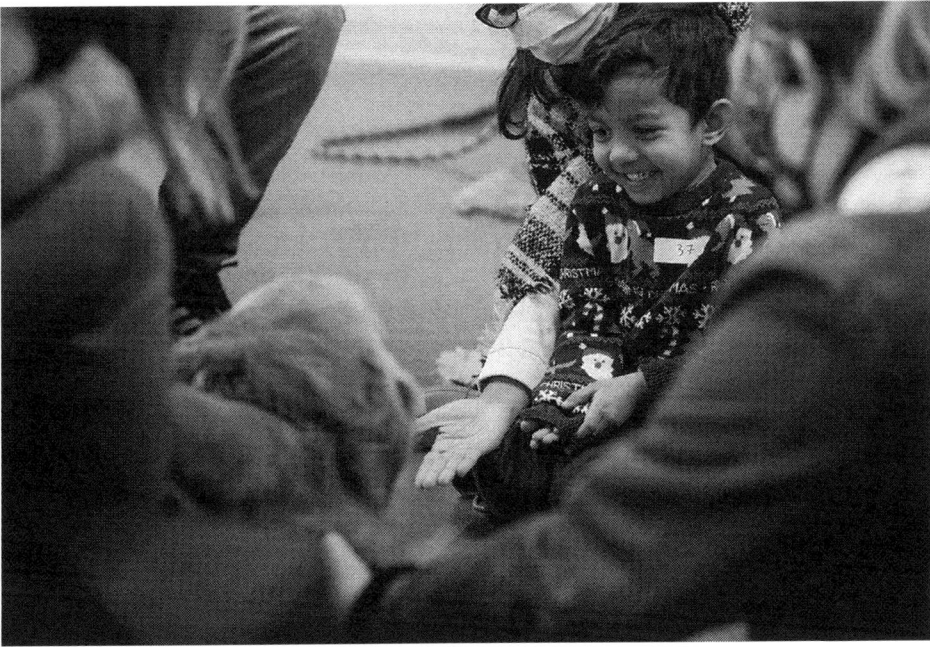

Figure 5.3 A mother modeling to her child how to obtain consent from a therapy dog

Source: Adam Lauzé – Sarah Lauzé Photography

Animal Welfare and Wildlife

Our attempts to define animal welfare within the context of AAIs fall short when we consider welfare with regards to wildlife. Interactions with wildlife vary enormously and range from zoo feeding programs that see visitors participate in the routine feeding of captive wildlife, to role-reversed safaris that see humans protected in cages to view wildlife, to the passive livestream viewing of birds at feeders. In our opening scenario in which food was left in a forest and wildlife filmed on a trail cam, we saw the natural behaviour of wildlife manipulated for human viewing pleasure. We might define welfare within the context of human-wildlife interactions as safeguarded by the following guiding principles:

1. No manipulative agents such as food or fencing are used to facilitate interactions.
2. Wildlife is viewed from a distance, and this distance is sufficient so as to not incite fear or suppress natural behaviours.
3. Within a virtual context, the use of discreet technology (i.e., a trail cam) that does not interfere with the display of natural behaviours is recommended.

Readers may be quick to point out an inconsistency here in the application of these principles and the opening scenario from Chapter 3 that saw Pat, a senior citizen in a residential home enjoy livestream video of a wild bird feeder. Isn't food within this context a manipulative agent and akin to the pizza left in the forest in this chapter's opening scenario? The use of food certainly is a recurring theme within both in-person and VHAIs, and we recognize there are readers who will take exception with the use of food in both the scenario found in Chapter 3 and the scenario for this chapter. In both instances, the natural behaviour of wildlife is manipulated – perhaps in the wild bird feeder less intrusively than the pizza-in-the-forest scenario – yet still manipulated. Tipping the scales in favor of the use of wild bird feeders is endorsement from the National Audubon Society (2023), which provides guidelines for the ethical feeding of wild birds that include stipulations around the content placed in feeders and the sanitary maintenance of feeders (see their guide here: www.audubon.org/news/to-feed-or-not-feed). Revisiting our definition of animal welfare for wildlife, we see that, within the context of HAIs, wildlife welfare is ensuring that wild animals' behaviour is not manipulated for the benefit of humans, free of coercion, fear, and direct human contact, and within a virtual context, facilitated via nonintrusive technology.

Repositioning the Animal as a Therapeutic Partner

It should also be emphasized that not every dog – or guinea pig, for that matter – is likely to be temperamentally suited to the role of therapy animal. By repeatedly obliging such animals to engage in uninvited social interactions with unfamiliar humans, some of whom may be very young or old, or abnormal in their behavior or demeanor, AAIs certainly have the potential to be highly stressful for the animal participants.

(Serpell et al., 2017, p. 228)

Safeguarding animal welfare is a necessary but insufficient condition supporting optimal HAI. Animals participating in AAIs whose welfare has been compromised engage clients less robustly and earnestly than do animals who willingly and, without coercion, invite clients to interact. There have been recent calls to reposition the animals working in AAIs as "therapeutic

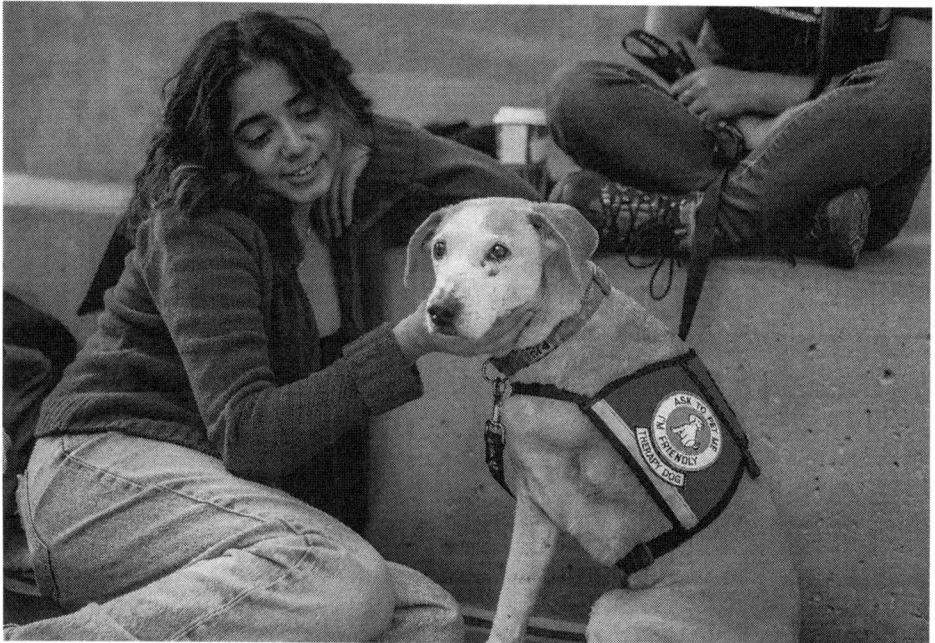

Figure 5.4 Student and therapy dog Craig interacting

Source: F. L. L. Green Photography

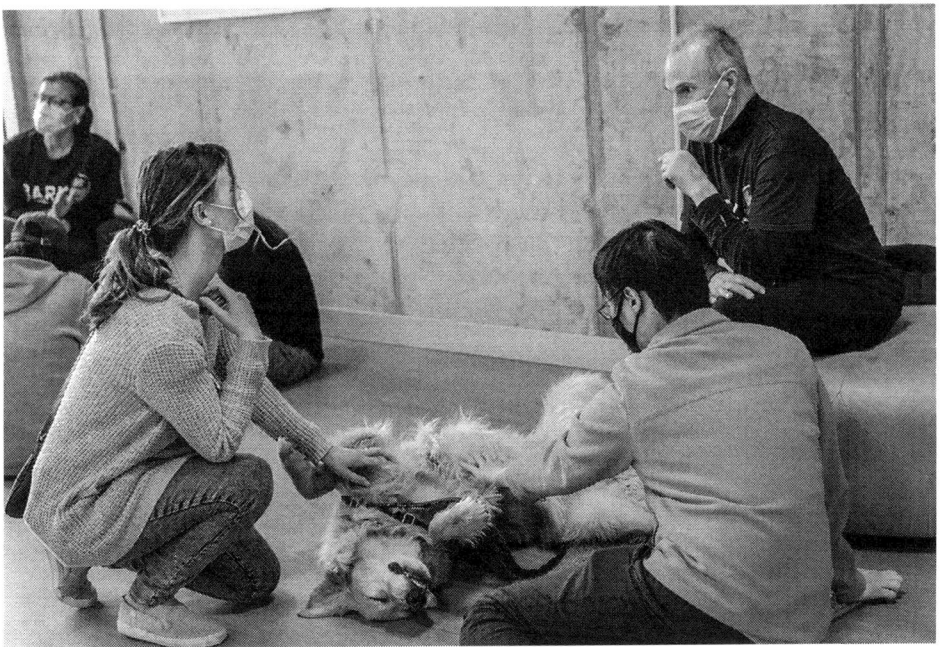

Figure 5.5 Therapy dog Doogle enjoying a session
Source: F. L. L. Green Photography

partners" – key agents in the very intervention designed to foster well-being outcomes in human participants (Collica-Cox & Day, 2021; Glenk & Foltin, 2021).

Glenk and Foltin (2021) argue that the animal's welfare is linked to the recipient's (or client's) welfare. Echoing the previous argument, when animal welfare is safeguarded within the context of AAI, the potential impact of the intervention itself is optimized (Mignot et al., 2022; Sarrafchi et al., 2022). Conversely, compromised animal welfare dilutes the effectiveness of the AAI. Thus, HAI researchers must take steps to ensure that the welfare of animals participating in AAIs is safeguarded and report incidences of compromised welfare as a factor impacting outcome effects. Safeguarding animal welfare within AAIs, above and beyond researchers' ethical responsibility, also contributes to empirical rigor. Fine and Chastain Griffin (2022) postulate that: "The outcome of the therapeutic intervention would not be relevant if the animals being engaged were not allowed to thrive" (p. 10). This assertion mirrors the call by researchers including Ng and colleagues (2015) who assert that animals working in AAI must flourish.

The Need for the Ongoing Monitoring of Animal Welfare

Many animal-handler teams undergo an initial screening and assessment process in order to be accepted as program volunteers, and although this is a critical step in ensuring that animals and handlers are well-suited to AAI-related work, it is but an initial step that must be supplemented with renewed certification and the ongoing monitoring of the team's abilities and animal welfare within sessions (Binfet & Hartwig, 2020). As therapy animals age, their ability to withstand the stressors inherent in AAIs diminishes, and this is an important consideration when including animals as part of AAI programming and research. The constant monitoring of animal welfare/

well-being throughout the AAI is key to ensuring animals are willingly participating and their wel-fare is not compromised. As argued by Ng et al. (2015), "We must continually measure animals' well-being and develop methods that can be applied to determine fatigue and stress" (p. 358). This invites the question: "Whose responsibility is it to monitor therapy animal welfare during AAIs?"

Glenk and Foltin (2021) describe handlers as having "split roles" – they must concomitantly monitor and manage the environment, guide their animal's behaviour, monitor their animal's welfare, and meet the needs of visiting clients. In short, this is no small undertaking, and this is particularly the case in virtual contexts as we will discuss in Chapter 6. Ideally, programs would have a "welfare monitor" whose sole task is to monitor, within sessions, animal welfare. This, of course, requires resources, and the reality is that many HAI programs, especially those posi-tioned as grassroots community organizations, do not have the ability to support this position. As a result, the responsibility falls largely on the handler to monitor the animal's well-being. This, however, is not without complications. In their call for best practices in canine-assisted interventions in hospital settings, Barker and Gee (2021) argue:

> The handler carries a heavy responsibility in monitoring their dog, their interactions with humans, and any potential risks in the environment. It is important for the CAI program and hospital to provide education and support to handlers in carrying out these responsibilities.
>
> (p. 5)

As has been addressed in the literature, concerns have been raised about the potential biases of both handlers and researchers regarding possible oversights around animal welfare. "People working within the AAA/AAT field may have a personal and biased perception that animals enjoy the interactions as much as the human participants" (Ng et al., 2015, p. 361). Handlers, for example, may be reluctant to report welfare issues for fear of repercussions from the animal therapy agency (i.e., curtailing of participation in sessions).

Within a research context, researchers must manage their biases too. Griffin and colleagues (2011) draw attention to researcher bias in the following description: "HAI (human-animal interaction) research tends to be conducted by animal lovers, who may be biased toward finding positive HAI effects" (p.6). Compromised animal welfare during an AAI can raise a whole host of challenges for researchers including, but not limited to, diluting the robustness of the AAI itself and, thereby, compromising potential findings and the posing of possible safety risks to human participants. Relatedly, researchers may be reluctant to halt an intervention that is under-way due to issues of animal welfare as on-the-spot solutions must be found (e.g., withdrawing an animal-handler team and finding a replacement team on short notice). Applied AAI research is a complicated undertaking and one that involves multiple stakeholders (e.g., therapy animals, clients, program staff, and researchers) working in, oftentimes, busy and complex settings (e.g., hospitals, open or shared spaces on a college campus). Animal welfare is a key element impact-ing the safety and engagement of all parties.

The Importance of Reporting Animal Safety and Well-Being in Research

Researchers conducting AAI studies to ascertain the effects on humans arising from interacting with therapy animals should report on the following:

1. That animal research ethics approval was obtained and report the certificate number;
2. How the welfare of animals was safeguarded throughout the research process, by whom, and with what qualifications;

3. Any incidents of animal distress or compromised well-being; and
4. Any incidents where safety was breeched, including a description.

In addition to this being important for animal welfare (i.e., holding researchers to account in upholding animal welfare protocols), the reporting of this information is important from an empirical perspective as mentioned earlier. Animals whose welfare is compromised during interventions comprising an AAI will engage human participants less effectively than would animals whose well-being was safeguarded as part of the intervention. This reflects one dimension of the study's implementation fidelity – was the intervention (i.e., the independent variable) administered as it was intended. Compromised animal welfare impacts the effectiveness of the HAI – the mechanism at the heart of the scientific investigation.

Factors Safeguarding Animal Welfare in Animal-Assisted Interventions

Training and Formation of Handlers

One aspect or dimension of an AAI that enhances optimal animal welfare is the comprehensive training of handlers. As highlighted earlier in this chapter, handlers have roles comprised of multiple tasks, and their primary task is to oversee their animal's welfare and well-being. It has been argued that handlers should adopt a proactive approach to managing their animal in public spaces where AAIs occur (Binfet & Hartwig, 2020). That is, handlers should anticipate factors that might compromise their animal's welfare. This might include verifying the working space is free of any noxious substances (e.g., food or dropped medication, positioning the animal

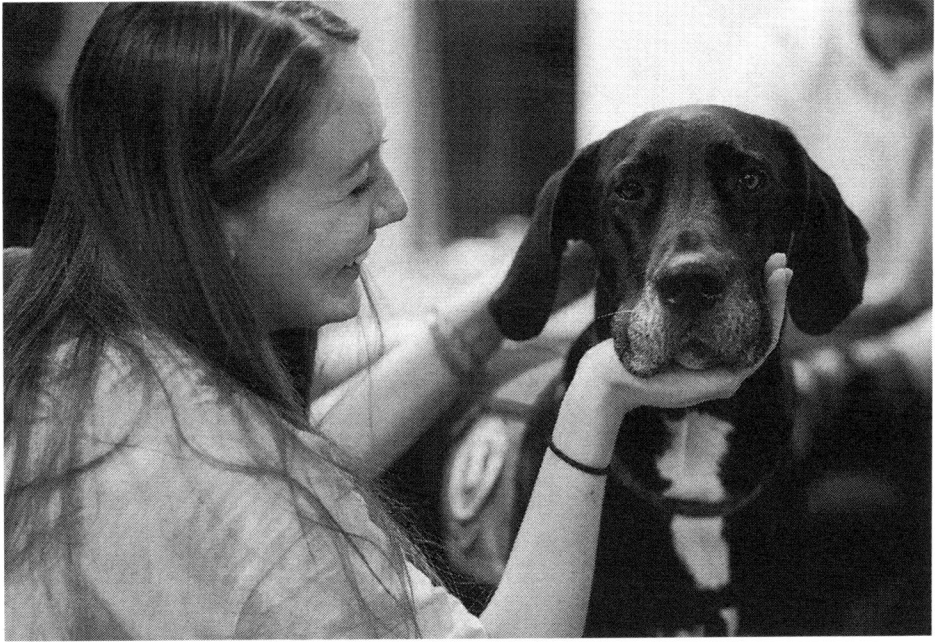

Figure 5.6 Student uses underhand pet after obtaining consent with therapy dog Layla

Source: Adam Lauzé – Sarah Lauzé Photography

in a way to minimize outside distractions, or curtailing overly enthusiastic human visitors to sessions). For an overview of research on dog-handler-client interactions and the intricacies faced by handlers participating in animal-assisted activities (AAA), see the recent publication by Roma and colleagues (2021).

Handlers must also facilitate or negotiate the interaction between their animal and the visiting client(s). This, in and of itself, is no small feat and requires ample social and emotional skills on the part of the handler (e.g., recognizing and managing their emotions, perspective-taking to understand clients' viewpoints). Key to facilitating this interaction is the education of the client as handlers bear the brunt of the responsibility around client education. This might include educating the client around how best to approach an animal, how to obtain consent from the animal, and behaviours to avoid that compromise the animal's well-being. The more clients are informed and educated around how best to interact with animals, the greater the likelihood that the HAI will be a rewarding experience for all stakeholders (i.e., the handler, the animal, the client) and the therapeutic animal partner's welfare safeguarded.

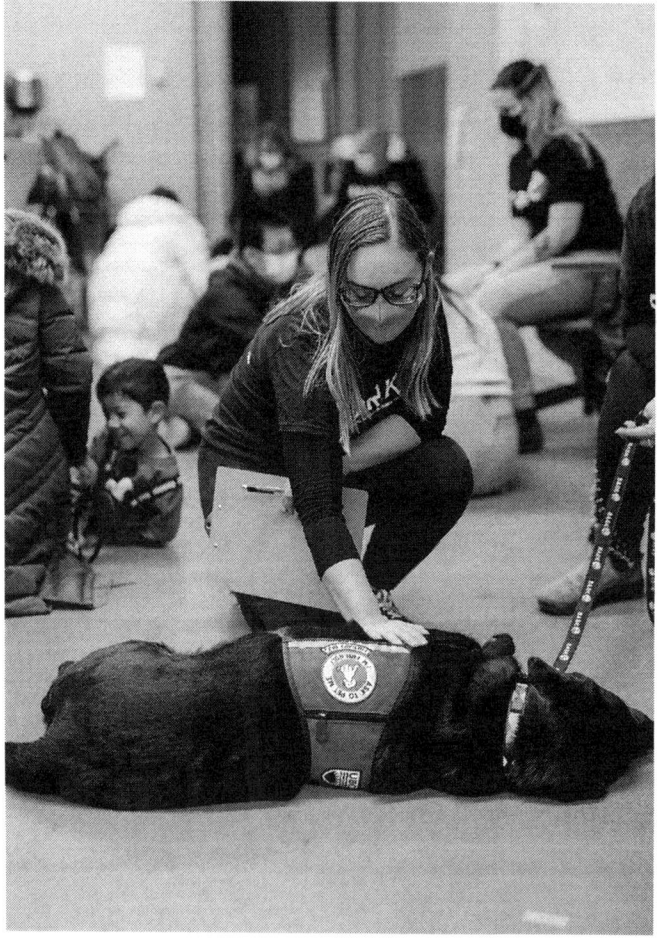

Figure 5.7 Program personnel monitoring canine well-being within a session

Source: Adam Lauzé – Sarah Lauzé Photography

Though this will vary from HAI program to program, handlers also bear a responsibility to identify clients in distress or who may need additional therapeutic support beyond the scope of an AAI. Recognizing that AAIs are considered an adjunct or complementary intervention (i.e., not an intervention providing counseling support to clients in need; Nepps et al., 2014; Nimer & Lundahl, 2007; Rossetti & King, 2010), participating in AAIs may heighten the emotions of clients and, in turn, result in clients disclosing information signaling that additional therapeutic support is warranted. As an illustration of this, handlers working in an on-campus canine-assisted intervention supporting college students' stress reduction might receive training on how to redirect students revealing thoughts of self-harm to the on-campus student support services/counselling office.

It perhaps goes without saying, but handlers must receive training around the identification of indicators of distress in the animals with whom they work. That is, as part of their training, handlers must receive species-specific education on the signs of distress common in their animal. As we've recognized in this chapter, ideally program personnel should assist with the monitoring of animal welfare, but the reality is that, oftentimes, such personnel is unavailable and responsibility of monitoring welfare rests solely with the handler. At the outset of this chapter, the research of Gut et al. (2018) was referenced as an illustration of an AAI where guinea pigs were the therapeutic partner. Common with guinea pigs is a *freezing* behaviour to indicate elevated fear, which sees the animal stop suddenly and remain motionless. Researchers and clients working with guinea pigs must be informed of this and other behaviours indicating that welfare has been compromised. Moreover, the training of the handler and the education of the visiting client must include information around how to proactively ensure that guinea pigs working in AAIs do not experience conditions that would result in a freezing response.

Emotional State Matching Between Handlers and Animals

The emotional state of the handler warrants discussion as this, too, can be a factor impacting their animal's welfare.

> Dogs are sensitive to their handlers' emotional states (Muller et al., 2015), and emotional contagion between owners and handlers is possible (Yong & Ruffman, 2014) contributing to the level of emotional disturbance experienced. Thus, dogs may mirror the anxiety and negative experiences of handlers in their cortisol levels, and this could actually happen in the context of AAA, as therapeutic work affects handler-dog teams who work in animal-assisted health care service both emotionally and physiologically (Kirchengast & Haubenhofer, 2007).
>
> (Pirrone et al., 2017, p. 51)

Within varied fields of study (i.e., education, psychology, medicine), the notion of emotional state matching or emotional contagion has gained increased attention as a factor impacting client or patient outcomes. For example, within education this might see a teacher with elevated stress influencing students' cortisol levels (Oberle & Schonert-Reichl, 2016) or healthcare providers' stress negatively influencing patients (Petitta et al., 2016). "Emotional contagion (EC) is the tendency to automatically mimic and synchronize the facial expressions, vocalizations, postures, and movements of the people we interact with (Hatfield et al., 1994)" (Petitta et al., 2016, p. 358). Within the context of AAIs, research is emerging that examines the notion of emotional contagion between handlers and their therapy animals. In a recent study by Silas and colleagues (2019), in a sample of 40 dog-handler teams, 25% of the handlers with elevated self-reports of

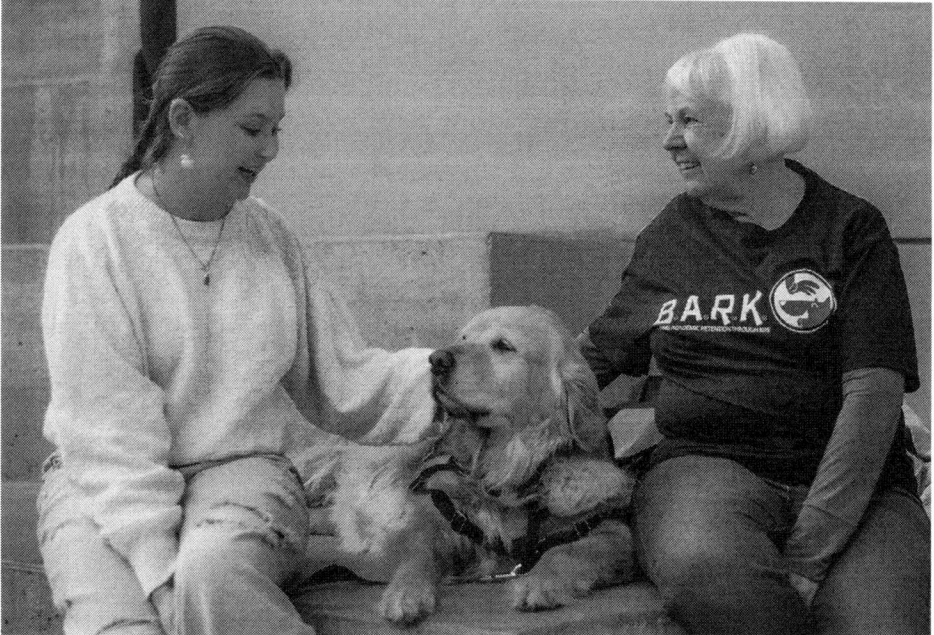

Figure 5.8 Handler Maureen facilitates visit between student and therapy dog Dash

Source: F. L. L. Green Photography

stress had dogs characterized by heightened stress. It was posited that handlers who themselves are characterized by heightened stress run the risk of transmitting stress to their dogs. These findings are in alignment with other HAI research that found participation in AAI potentially stressful for therapy dogs (e.g., Sarrafchi et al., 2022; Uccheddu et al., 2018).

Visitor Education/Instruction Key to Reducing Animal Stress During Sessions

A key element or dimension of in-person AAIs that help safeguard animal welfare within sessions is the education or instruction given to human clients seeking to interact with animals. Falling on the shoulders of program administrators or, oftentimes, the handlers themselves, instructions to visiting clients on how to optimally interact with an animal can reduce the likelihood of interactions compromising animal welfare. Ideally, this information would be shared with clients prior to the session; however, the reality of many programs is they may be delivered in public spaces without clients preregistering for a session. There is, thus, little opportunity to instruct clients on how best to interact with animals participating in an AAI, and the responsibility then falls on the handler to establish guidelines with the client upon their arrival to a session. This is especially the case during on-campus therapy dog programs that see interest from students typically surpass the program's capacity to meet the needs of all the students seeking to interact with dogs.

The challenges are different, of course, within the context of VHAIs where there is no physical interaction between the visitor and the animal. Rather, the challenge becomes creating opportunities for the visitor to become engaged in the interaction. This might take the form of the handler sharing information about the animal in question and inviting the client to ask questions about the animal or to guide the client through a simulation session (e.g., "Imagine you are here with us in the room and you're petting the dog from the top of his forehead back toward his tail").

Factors Compromising Animal Welfare in Human-Animal Interactions

Dogs working in HAI (i.e., animal-assisted activities/therapy/coaching/education), and varied species more generally, may have their welfare compromised by the duration of sessions, the frequency of sessions, and the number of clients supported during a session (King et al., 2011; Marinelli et al., 2009). Certainly, there is a risk of this in on-campus canine-visitation stress-reduction programs or canine-assisted interventions where the interest of college students to spend time with therapy dogs often surpasses the program's capacity to provide opportunities for interactions. Limiting the duration of individual sessions, the number of sessions per week in which animal-handler teams participate, the number of new environments animals are required to adapt to, and the number and behaviour of clients/visitors supported are all factors that can individually and collectively compromise therapy animal welfare (see Table 5.1 for a welfare checklist for animals participating in virtual human-animal interactions).

Animal Welfare in Virtual Human-Animal Interactions

Challenges to Animal Welfare Within a Virtual Context

Just like in-person AAI sessions that see therapy animals and their handlers face challenges that can compromise animal welfare, so, too, are there challenges within a virtual context. In an in-person context, we might see the welfare of animals compromised by the stress associated with working in close proximity to other animals, challenges around adapting to a new environment, and challenges associated with the type and number of clients supported. Within a virtual context, we might see challenges around the handler having to organize all aspects of filming while concurrently monitoring their animal's well-being including the troubleshooting of technological difficulties, an issue which we discuss again in the next chapter. The handler must deal with several challenges including: heat from additional lighting, challenges related to capturing audio, the challenge of keeping the animal within the viewing frame when filming, challenges related to following a script or consulting a bank of questions if a part of the protocol, and, if synchronously delivered, the challenge of responding to clients and their questions in real-time (e.g., responding to Zoom chat questions). As can be imagined, there is no shortage of potential obstacles or challenges that individually and collectively can undermine and thwart the welfare of animals participating in AAIs. Handler training or practice sessions where handlers and their animals can become familiar with technology and the filming studio/space can help reduce welfare risks, thereby helping ensure that animal-handler teams are comfortable and can optimally engage with viewers/clients. Having program personnel who can assist with technology, provide prompts to help the handler remain on script, and monitor animal welfare can reduce the burden of tasks on the shoulders of the handler and help ensure animal well-being during virtual sessions. We discuss each of these points in more detail in the next chapter.

Benefits and Limitations of Virtual Human-Animal Interactions to Animal Welfare

Virtual Interactions a Potential Buffer to Animal Stress?

Might virtual AAI reduce wear and tear on animals and thereby safeguard their well-being? That is, there is no direct animal-to-client contact, reducing the potential stress arising from hands-on interactions. Though perhaps not as demanding on the animal as in-person sessions, virtual AAIs can be a taxing undertaking for animals, especially as they age. Though there are no demands to physically engage with clients, animals working in virtual AAIs must often hold steady their position for prolonged periods to remain within the viewing frame. Oftentimes too, animals working indoors might be on an elevated platform that allows the handler to be at their level and this poses a potential challenge for older animals unaccustomed to this workspace arrangement. Veteran therapy animals accustomed to interacting with clients or the public may have difficulty adjusting to the less robust interactions of a VHAI session that, oftentimes, sees them remain rather static and only interact with their handler.

An additional benefit arising from VHAIs is that the animal-handler team can remain in their home environment and prerecord or film live from the location of their choosing (i.e., a location where the animal is most comfortable). This, in turn, reduces the stress of the animal adapting to a new and unfamiliar environment. As recognized by Ein et al. (2022): "These virtual AAIs can protect the wellbeing of the animal given the possibility that the animal may not always enjoy being involved in these interventions" (p. 16).

Recognize that there might be limitations for the animals working in VHAI contexts that see them miss out on opportunities to receive affection, form new bonds, and to possibly socialize with other animals. Relatedly, the handlers who may be motivated to volunteer in AAI programming to meet socializing needs (Rousseau et al., 2020) may find virtual interactions less satisfying in meeting their needs.

Conclusion

In this chapter, we defined animal welfare within the context of HAI/AAI and identified factors safeguarding and undermining welfare. Our definition of animal welfare is broadly informed by the Five Freedoms and incorporates considerations of animal consent, relationship-driven handler practices, and opportunities for animals, as part of their interaction, to demonstrate natural behaviours that reflect them flourishing within their assigned environment. Our definition of welfare was examined within the context of wildlife interactions and considerations for welfare within virtual contexts were discussed. We turn next to a discussion of creating and actualizing virtual human-animal connections.

Table 5.1 Welfare Checklist: Considerations for Animals Participating in Virtual Human-Animal Interactions

1. Have the animal and handler undergone screening to determine suitability for the work in question? (i.e., has the animal's potential to participate in virtual human-animal connections been assessed?)
2. If supplemental lighting is used to support the quality of filming, is the temperature being monitored to prevent animals overheating?
3. Is water available before, during, and after filming?
4. Has the human participant been provided instruction/education regarding how to optimally interact?
5. Have efforts been made to obtain consent from the animal?
6. Does the interaction encourage the animal to demonstrate natural behaviours?
7. Is the animal determining participation and able to voluntarily cease to participate?
8. Is the duration of the intervention and the number of interventions per day in accordance with recommended best practices?
9. Have time-out breaks been scheduled as part of each working session?
10. Have barriers or deterrents to reporting adverse effects been acknowledged/recognized? (i.e., reflecting poorly on the agency)
11. Is there a designated human responsible for the welfare advocacy of the animal? If not, how will the handler monitor welfare whilst concurrently overseeing the virtual human-animal interaction session?

References

Ace Vlogs. (2023). *What happens to a pizza left in the woods?* [Video]. *YouTube*. www.youtube.com/watch?v=19VgS-CeGCQ

Barker, S. B., & Gee, N. R. (2021). Canine-assisted interventions in hospitals: Best practices for maximizing human and canine safety. *Frontiers in Veterinary Science, 8*, 1–12. https://doi.org/10.2289/fvets.2021.615730

Binfet, J. T., & Hartwig, E. (2020). *Canine assisted interventions: A comprehensive guide to credentialing therapy dog teams.* New York: Routledge. https://doi.org/10.4324/9780429436055

Broom, D. (1986). Indicators of poor welfare. *British Veterinary Journal, 142*, 524–526. https://doi.org/10.1016.0007-1935(86)90109-0

Collica-Cox, K., & Day, G. J. (2021). Dogs as therapeutic partners, not therapeutic tools: Ethical considerations for AAT in correctional settings. *Social Sciences, 10*, 432. https://doi.org/10.3390/socsci10110432

De Santis, M., Contalbrigo, L., Borgi, M., Cirulli, F., Luzi, F., . . . Farina, L. (2017). Equine assisted interventions (EAIs): Methodological considerations for stress assessment in horses. *Veterinary Sciences, 4*(3), 44. https://doi.org/1-.3390/vetsci4030044

Ein, N., Gervasio, J., Reed, M. J., & Vickers, K. (2022). Effects of exposure to dog videos before a stress. *Anthrozoos*. https://doi.org/10.1080/08927936.2022.2149925

Fine, A. H., & Chastain Griffin, T. (2022). Protecting animal welfare in animal-assisted interventions: Our ethical obligation. *Seminars in Speech and Language, 43*(1), 8–23. https://doi.org/10.1055/s-0441-1742099

Fry, N. E. (2021). Welfare considerations for horses in therapy and education services. In J. M. Peralta & A. H. Fine (Eds.), *The welfare of animals in animal-assisted interventions: Foundations and best practice methods* (pp. 219–242). Springer Nature. https://doi.org/10.1007/978-3-030-69587-3_9

Glenk, L. M. (2017). Current perspectives on therapy dog welfare in animal-assisted interventions. *Animals, 7*(7), 1–17. Https://doi.org/10.3390/ani7020007

Glenk, L. M., & Foltin, S. (2021). Therapy dog welfare revisited: A review of the literature. *Veterinary Sciences, 8*(10), 226–244. https://doi.org/10.3390/vetsci8100226

Griffin, J. A., McCune, S., Malhomes, V., & Hurley, K. (2011). Human-animal interaction research: An introduction to issues and topics. In P. McCarle, S. McCune, J. A. Griffin, & V. Maholmes (Eds.), How animals affect us: Examining the influence of human-animal interaction on child development and human health (pp. 3–9). American Psychological Association.

Gut, W., Crump, L., Zinsstag, J., Hattendorf, J., & Hediger, K. (2018). The effect of human interaction on guinea pig behavior in animal-assisted therapy. Journal of Veterinary Behavior, 25, 56–64.

Hatch, A. (2007). The view from all fours: A look at an animal-assisted activity program from the animal's perspective. *Anthrozoös, 20*, 37–50.

Hatfield, E., Cacioppo, J. T., & Rapson, R. L. (1994). *Emotional contagion.* Cambridge University Press.

Hetts, S., Clark, J. D., Arnold, C. E., & Mateo, J. M. (1992). Influence of housing conditions on beagle behaviour. *Applied Animal Behaviour Science, 61*, 63–77.

Horrowitz, A. (2021). Considering the "dog" in dog-human interaction. *Frontiers in Veterinary Science, 8*, 1–5. https://doi.org/10.3389/fvets.2021.642821

Howe, R., & Kroll, T. (2022). Why should the welfare of therapy animals involved in animal assisted interventions matter to child healthcare researchers and professionals? *Comprehensive Child and Adolescent Nursing, 45*(2), 123–126. https://doi.org/10.1080/24694193.2022.2060377

International Association of Human-Animal Interaction Organizations. (2018). *IAHAIO White Paper.* Retrieved January 3, 2023, from http://iahaio.org/wp/wpcontent/uploads/2018/04/iahaio_wp_updated-2018-final.pdf

King, C., Watters, J., & Mungre, S. (2011). Effect of a time-out session with working animal-assisted therapy dogs. *Journal of Veterinary Behavior: Clinical Applications and Research, 6*, 232–238.

Kirchengast, S., & Haubenhofer, D. K. (2007). Dog handlers and dogs emotional and cortisol secretion responses associated with animal-assisted therapy sessions. *Society & Animals, 15*, 127–150.

Marinelli, L., Normando, S., Siliprandi, C., Salvadoretti, M., & Mongillo, P. (2009). Dog assisted interventions in a specialized centre and potential concerns for animal welfare. *Veterinary Research Communication, 33*, 93–95.

McBride, E. A., & Baugh, S. (2022). Animal welfare in context: Historical, scientific, ethical, moral and One welfare perspectives. In A. Vitale & S. Pollo (Eds.), *Human/animal relationships in transformation* (pp. 119–147). The Palgrave Macmillan Animal Ethics Series.

Mellor, D. J. (2017). Operational details of the Five Domani Model and its key applications to the assessment and management of animal welfare. *Animals, 7*(8), 60. https://doi/org/10.3390/ani70800600

Mignot, A., de Luca, K., Servais, V., & Leboucher, G. (2022). Handler's representations on therapy dog welfare. *Animals, 580,* 1–11. https://doi.org/10.3390/ani12050580

Muller, C. A., Schmitt, K., Barber, A. L., & Huber, L. (2015). Dogs can discriminate emotional expressions of human faces. *Current Biology, 25,* 601–605. https://doi.org/10.1016/jcub.2014.12.055

Muvhali, P. T. (2018). *Improving ostrich welfare by developing positive human-animal interactions* [Master's thesis, University of StellenBosch].

National Audubon Society. (2023). *To feed, or not to feed: Backyard feeders are good for birds, as long as you follow these simple rules.* Retrieved January 10, 2023 from www.audubon.org/news/to-feed-or-not-feed

Nepps, P., Stewart, C. N., & Bruckno, S. R. (2014). Animal-assisted activity: Effects of a complementary intervention program on psychological and physiological variables. *Journal of Evidence Based Complementary Alternative Medicine, 19*(3), 211–215. https://doi.org/10.1177/2156587214533570

Ng, Z., Albright, J., Fine, A. H., & Peralta, J. (2015). Our ethical and moral responsibility: Ensuring the welfare of therapy animals. In A. Fine (Ed.), *Handbook on animal-assisted therapy* (4th ed., pp. 357–376). Elsevier.

Ng, Z. Y., Morse, L., Albright, J., Viera, A., & Souza, M. (2019). Describing the use of animals in animal-assisted intervention research. *Journal of Applied Animal Welfare Science, 22,* 364–376. https://doi.org/10.1080/10888705.2018.1524765

Nimer, J., & Lundahl, B. (2007, September). Animal-assisted therapy: A meta-analysis. *Anthrozoös, 20*(3), 225–238.

Novak, M. A., & Drewsen, K. H. (1989). Enriching the lives of captive primates: Issues and problems. In E. F. Segal (Ed.), *Housing, care, and psychological wellbeing of captive and laboratory primates* (pp. 161–185). Noyes.

Nussbaum, M., & Sen, A. (2004). *The quality of life.* Routledge.

Oberle, E., & Schonert-Reichl, K. A. (2016). Stress contagion in the classroom? The link between classroom teacher burnout and morning cortisol in elementary school students. *Social Science & Medicine, 159,* 30–37. https://doi.org/10.1016/j.socscimed.2016.04.031

Overall, K. L. (2013, September 1). *Fear factor: Is routine veterinary care contributing to lifelong patient anxiety?* Retrieved from http://veterinarynews.dvm360.com/fear-factor-routine-veterinary-care-contributing-lifelong-patient-anxiety

Pet Partners. (2018). *Standards of practice in animal-assisted interventions.* Retrieved January 3, 2023, from https://petpartners.org/standards/

Petitta, L., Jiang, L., & Hartel, C. E. J. (2016). Emotional contagion and burnout among nurses and doctors: Do joy and anger from different sources of stakeholders matter? *Stress & Health, 33*(4), 358–369.

Pirrone, F., Ripamonti, A., Garoni, E. C., Stradiotti, S., & Albertini, M. (2017). Measuring social synchrony and stress in the handler-dog dyad during animal-assisted activities: A pilot study. *Journal of Veterinary Behavior, 21,* 45–52. https://doi.org/10.1016/j.jveb.2017.07.004.

Roma, R. P. S., Tardif-Williams, C. Y., Moore, S. A., & Bosacki, S. L. (2021). A transdisciplinary perspective on dog-handler client interactions in animal assisted activities for children, youth, and young adults. *Human-Animal Interaction Bulletin, 9*(2), 62–91.

Rossetti, J., & King, C. (2010). Use of animal-assisted therapy with psychiatric patients: A literature review. *Journal of Psychosocial Nursing and Mental Health Services, 48*(11), 44–48.

Rousseau, C. X., Binfet, J. T., Green, F. L. L., Tardif-Williams, C., Draper, Z., & Maynard, A. (2020). Up the leash: An investigation of handler well-being and perceptions of volunteering in canine-assisted interventions. *Pet Behavior Science, 10,* 15–35. https://doi.org/10.2107/pbs.vi10.12598I

Sarrafchi, A., David-Steel, M., Pearce, S. D., & de Zwaan, N. (2022). Effect of human-dog interaction on therapy dog stress during an on-campus student stress buster event. *Applied Animal Behaviour Science, 253.* https://doi.org/10.1016/j.applanim.2022.105659

Scalia, B., Alberghina, D., & Panzera, M. (2017). Influence of low stress handling during clinical visit on physiological and behavioural indicators in adult dogs: A preliminary study. *Pet Behaviour Science*, *4*, 20–22. doi: 10.21071/pbs.v0i4.10131

Serpell, J., McCune, S., Gee, N., & Griffin, J. A. (2017). Current challenges to research on animal-assisted interventions. *Applied Developmental Science*, *21*(3), 223–233. http://dx.doi.org/10.1080/10888691.20 16.1262775

Silas, H. J., Binfet, J. T., & Ford, A. T. (2019). Therapeutic for all? Observational assessments of therapy canine stress in an on-campus stress-reduction program. *Journal of Veterinary Behavior*, *32*, 6–13. Https://doi.org/10.1016/j.jveb.2019.03.009

Uccheddu, S., Albertini, M., Pierantoni, L., Fantino, S., & Pirrone, F. (2018). Assessing behavior and stress in two dogs during sessions of a reading-to-a-dog program for children with pervasive developmental disorders. *Dog Behavior*, *4*, 1–12. https://dx.doi.org/10.4454/db.v4i3.83

Wagner, C., Grob, C., & Hediger, K. (2022). Specific and non-specific factors of animal-assisted interventions considered in research: A systematic review. *Frontiers in Psychology*, 158103. Https://www.crd.york.ac.uk/prospero/display_record.php?

Webster, J. (1994). *Animal welfare: A cool eye towards Eden*. Blackwell.

Yin, S. (2009). *Low stress handling, restraint and behavior modification of dogs and cats: Techniques for patients who love their visits*. Cattle Dog Publishing.

Yong, M. H., & Ruffman, T. (2014). Emotional contagion: Dogs and humans show a similar physiological response to human infant crying. *Behavioural Processes*, *108*, 155–165. https://doi.org/10.1016/j.beproc.2014.10.006

6 Best Practices in Creating Virtual Human-Animal Connections

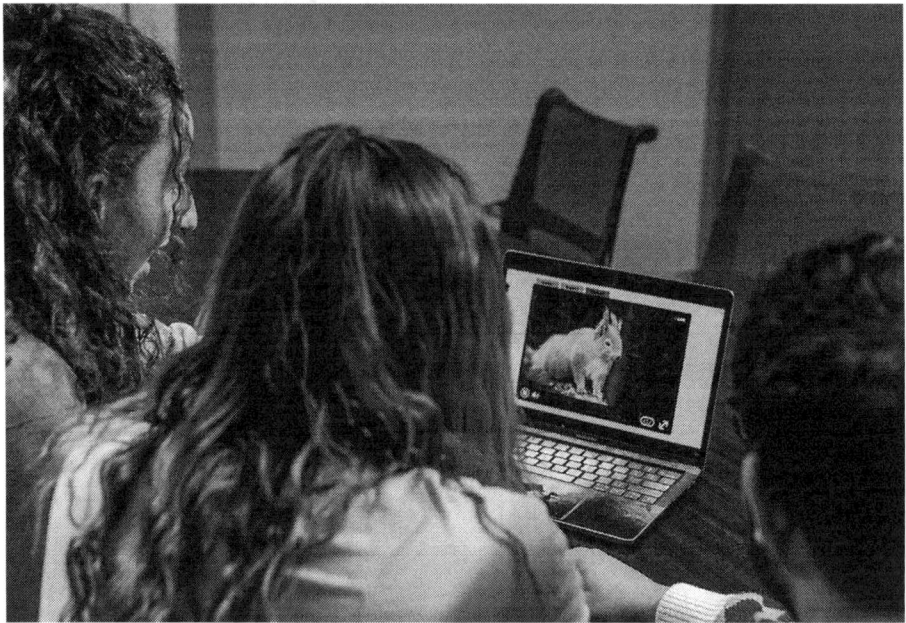

Figure 6.1 A group of students sitting at a table with a laptop watching a video of a squirrel in nature
Source: F. L. L. Green Photography

Scenario

I want to foster virtual human-animal connections in the classroom! But where do I start and what challenges will I encounter?

Mr. Bhatt has been teaching fourth grade for over ten years and is an animal lover who lives on a farm with two horses, four sheep, three cows, two dogs, two cats, and several chickens and rabbits. He has always included discussions about animals and principles of humane education as part of the curriculum because he believes that, as an elementary educator, he has a responsibility to teach children about animals' needs and how to respect their welfare. He relies mostly on traditional approaches to include animal-related content in the classroom, such as videos, storybooks, and discussions about animals. He recently talked to a colleague who took her fifth grade class to visit a donkey sanctuary, an experience that her students cherished deeply and

DOI: 10.4324/9781003327868-6

that fueled thoughtful in-class discussion about animal welfare. He is eager to offer a similar experience to his fourth grade students, but he knows that he will have to be creative and explore alternative strategies because some of his students are allergic to or fearful of different animals. Recently, he has been excited to learn about virtual therapy dogs and virtual zoo visits and animal livestreams. Mr. Bhatt is keen to explore how he might virtually connect his students and his beloved farm animals, but he wonders where to start and what challenges he'll encounter.

Questions for Reflection

1. What strategies could Mr. Bhatt use to virtually connect his students to animals including his beloved farm animals?
2. What are some of the preparatory and technological considerations involved in structuring virtual human-animal connections?
3. How can we engage participants in virtual human-animal connections?
4. How can we assess the benefits of virtual human-animal connections for participants?

Best Practices in Creating Virtual Human-Animal Connections

As the field of HAIs continues to expand, there is a growing interest in creating opportunities for people to virtually interact with animals. In this book, we have argued that VHAIs are one way to expand the field of HAIs and to reach a larger and more diverse group of learners, and we have considered various ways that people virtually connect with animals and have discussed some of the associated welfare considerations. In this chapter, we consider best practices in creating opportunities for virtual human-animal connections. Building on the foundational information shared thus far in our book, including our research developing virtual canine comfort modules (Binfet et al., 2022; Tardif-Williams et al., 2023), we deliver on our promise to offer tangible strategies around how best to design, structure, and deliver virtual human-animal connections. We address the mechanics of structuring VHAIs, including considerations of design and delivery; handler training and preparation; the use of scripts, technology, and videography; how to engage virtual viewers; and the assessment of the benefits of virtual human-animal connections on participants. We also provide a checklist for readers, offering them support and guidance in the creation and actualization of virtual human-animal connections (see Table 6.1).

Table 6.1 Checklist for Creating and Actualization of Virtual Human-Animal Connections

Steps in Creating and Actualizing VHAIs	*Key Factors to Consider*

Identifying the goals for creating VHAIs	What type of VHAIs do you want to create and *why*? What are your goals for creating and delivering VHAIs?
	• **Educational**
	  ○ Supporting people's reading or learning in other areas (e.g., math, employment-related knowledge)
	  ○ Increasing students' knowledge about animals' habitats, behaviours, and social and welfare needs
	• **Social connections and well-being**
	  ○ Facilitating social interactions
	  ○ Supporting well-being (e.g., reducing stress, anxiety, loneliness or homesickness, promoting positive affect and happiness)

(Continued)

Table 6.1 (Continued)

Steps in Creating and Actualizing VHAIs	Key Factors to Consider

Choosing the design and method of delivery of VHAIs	*How* will you create and deliver VHAIs? Will you create synchronous or asynchronous VHAIs? What social media platform will you utilize to deliver VHAIs? What is the platform and social media preference of your intended audience?
	• **Asynchronous or prerecorded platforms**
	  ◦ Well-suited to reaching a large and diverse audience of virtual viewers, can be accessed from any geographic location and at any time, and might be preferred by people who are socially shy or who feel marginalized, such as people within BIPOC and 2SLGBTQI+ communities
	• **Synchronous or live platforms**
	  ◦ Well-suited to reaching a diverse audience of virtual viewers, and might be preferred by people who are seeking to engage in real-time interactions with animals and social connections

Personnel needs	*Who* will you involve in the process of creating and delivering VHAIs? What expertise will you require? Who will join your team or supporting cast?
	• **Types of expertise**
	  ◦ Researchers and research assistants
	  ◦ Indigenous knowledge experts
	  ◦ Videographers
	  ◦ Photographers
	  ◦ Animal welfare monitors
	  ◦ Experienced dog handlers
	  ◦ Monitors to compile and address participants' questions during synchronous sessions
	  ◦ *Technology-confident hosts* to handle any technological challenges that arise
	  ◦ Video editor
	  ◦ Social media expert to assist with dissemination

Handler training and preparation	How will you train and prepare animal handlers for their role in creating and delivering VHAIs?
	• **Key steps to consider in handler training and preparation**
	  ◦ Technology training and support
	  ◦ A handler handbook (e.g., outlining etiquette and expectations, detailing key online programming prerequisites such as tips on how to use social media platforms, what platforms are popular)
	  ◦ A handler script (e.g., formal or semi-structured, guided mindfulness practice, animal-themed meditations)
	  ◦ Practice sessions to promote familiarization with the featured animal(s), the filming location or setting, and with the personnel including the videographer(s) and video equipment
	  ◦ Handler *telepresence-focused* training (e.g., using a clear tone-of-voice with more verbal affirmations and to be more deliberately overt in their facial expressions and body language.
	  ◦ Discussion about intensive time commitment and how to mitigate feeling overwhelmed
	  ◦ Negotiating plans to protect handlers' confidentiality

Table 6.1 (Continued)

Steps in Creating and Actualizing VHAIs	Key Factors to Consider

Navigating the animal's role	How will you navigate and prepare the animal(s) for their role in creating and delivering VHAIs?
	• **Key steps to consider in navigating the animal(s)' role**
	  ○ Screening animal(s) for suitability
	  ○ Practice sessions to promote familiarization with filming crew and equipment, new studio space or adjustments made to their familiar home-based context, unfamiliar visitors, and lighting and heat associated with filming
	  ○ Developing a protocol to monitor the animal(s) for signs of distress during all stages and appropriate action plan should a session be terminated due to signs of animal distress

Technology and videography	How will you create polished, professional videos or synchronous VHAIs?
	• **Key aspects to consider**
	  ○ Access to high-quality technology and a strong internet connection
	  ○ Length of VHAI session(s)
	  ○ Optimal filming conditions (e.g., lighting, camera angles, quiet and distraction-free environment, camera positioned at eye level and stabilized, comfortable room temperature for humans and animals)
	  ○ Access to *technology-confident hosts* available during the creation and delivery of VHAIs.
	  ○ Create a back-up contact plan in case there are technical difficulties (contact by email, text, or phone)
	  ○ Filming VHAIs
	  ○ Editing prerecorded VHAIs
	  ○ Dissemination of VHAIs

Engaging virtual viewers	How will you engage people in VHAIs?
	• **Key aspects to consider**
	  ○ Ensuring that your intended audience has access to technology and a strong internet connection, and that they know the procedure to follow should they encounter technical difficulties
	  ○ Offering *client education* on how to use the social media platform, the available time(s) and best location for accessing (i.e., quiet space) VHAIs, and what to expect during the VHAI session(s)
	  ○ Engaging people in animal-themed guided mindfulness meditations to promote virtual human-animal connections, a sense of *being there* or *being with others/featured animal(s)*
	  ○ Considering people's preferred length of VHAIs and social format (e.g., one-on-one or small group, familiar or unfamiliar group members)
	  ○ Providing more animal-specific information and creating more interactive VHAIs (e.g., involving the animal(s) in activities)
	  ○ Encouraging opportunities for authentic participatory experiences (e.g., giving the dog a treat or petting the cat via the handler as translator)

Assessing the impact of VHAIs on participants	How do you plan to assess the impact of VHAIs?
	• **Key aspects to consider**
	  ○ Formal assessments should include the use of standardized measures as determined in consultation with a researcher with expertise in the field of HAIs
	  ○ Informal assessments should consider the extent to which people participate, engage, and enjoy their virtual connections with animals
	  ○ Consideration to the complexity and diversity of people's virtual experiences with animals

Choosing the Design and Method of Delivery of Virtual Human-Animal Connections

A first consideration for researchers, educators, or professionals is identifying the goal for creating virtual human-animal connections and then choosing the best design and method of delivery. Recalling the scenario featured at the outset of this chapter, Mr. Bhatt will need to reflect on *why* he wants to virtually connect his students to animals (his goals for VHAIs), as this will inform *how* he proceeds in creating VHAIs for his students. As discussed in Chapter 4, educators and practitioners might want to incorporate virtual connections with animals, in combination with or in addition to mindfulness practice, as a way to help students and clients deal with stress and anxiety by grounding them firmly and restoratively in the present moment. Research supports the stress-relieving and mood-enhancing benefits of quietly observing animals via digital technologies (i.e., watching dogs, cats, birds and wildlife; Crowley et al., 2021; Ein et al., 2020, 2021, 2022; Kogan et al., 2018). Also, educators and practitioners might consider creating virtual connections with animals during classroom instruction or counselling sessions as a way to facilitate timely *brain breaks* – which can help people feel more relaxed physically and mentally and can enhance learning and engagement by increasing focus. Educators might be motivated to create VHAIs as a way to teach students about a diversity of animals and their habitats, behaviours, and social and welfare needs. Still, educators and practitioners might be motivated in harnessing the potential of VHAIs to support people's learning, reading, and employment-related knowledge; foster social connections; reduce stress, homesickness, and loneliness; and/ or promote feelings of happiness and well-being.

Once a goal for creating virtual human-animal connections has been established, a second consideration involves the design and method of delivery. Here, we glean insights from the research on virtual mental health services more generally, where we learn that there are important variations in the design of services and in the method of accessing remote support which must be considered (Barak & Grohol, 2011). Such variations can be partially explained by the goals of the interventions (Davies et al., 2014) and by the characteristics of the people (e.g., experience with and preference for online engagement). For example, some interventions aim to promote people's well-being or to prevent the experience of mental health challenges through self-access to standard content in blogs or to predefined modules with themes (e.g., management of stress) related to well-being (Day et al., 2013; Hintz et al., 2015). Other interventions follow the principles of standard theoretical approaches for in-person support (e.g., cognitive behavioural therapy) and involve professionally guided contact with a mental health professional (e.g., online counselling via Skype). Clearly, these differences in online mental health services shape the level of initiative required from the participant as well as the levels of inter-activity with technological resources and/or the direct connection with professionals involved in the programs.

Similarly, these differences must be considered when designing virtual human-animal supports and assessing the impact of virtual connections with animals on people's learning, social connections, or well-being. Depending on the goal for creating virtual human-animal connections, it might be better to consider a synchronous or asynchronous platform for design and delivery. For instance, if the goal is to foster social connections among isolated long-term care home residents or to deliver animal-assisted therapy to help a group of young people manage trauma-related experiences, then a synchronous platform might work best to facilitate weekly interactions among several residents and a therapy animal and handler. Rather, if the goal is to teach students about elephants' habitats, behaviours, and social and welfare needs, then a combination of a livestream webcam featuring elephants (including opportunities to engage in *elephant walks*) and YouTube videos featuring elephants in their natural habitats might equally spark critical discussions about elephants within the classroom setting. Educators might also be motivated to foster reading skills in their younger students in which case it might make sense to create virtual, synchronous opportunities to read stories to a dog. Other goals for creating VHAIs might include a counselling or therapeutic focus with people experiencing mental health challenges such as depression, anxiety, or post-traumatic stress disorder. In these latter cases, VHAIs might be best delivered as predefined modules that can be accessed asynchronously where people can engage in private, one-on-one, and self-paced virtual interactions with a therapy animal and handler.

Also, as noted before, there are important variations in the method of accessing online supports (Barak & Grohol, 2011), and such variations can be partially explained by people's characteristics (e.g., experience with and preference for online engagement, desire for social interaction). As such, it is equally important to consider people's preferred technology and social media platform when designing VHAIs (Fernandes et al., 2021). Some virtual viewers might prefer to engage using one of several asynchronous platforms (e.g., Facebook, Instagram) or via a synchronous platform (e.g., YouTube, Zoom). Given that the goal is to maximally engage people with animals in a virtual context, the first consideration should be the best method of delivery.

As research on VHAIs advances, we learn that much consideration goes into the creation of opportunities for virtual connections between people and animals. Here, we remind the reader that, as discussed in Chapter 4, educators and practitioners could leverage the potential of a range of existing and easily accessible digital technologies to create VHAIs and support people's learning, social connections, and well-being. These exciting digital technologies could include virtual reality and immersive experiences as well as a variety of content and contexts (e.g., live nest, trail, farm and underwater webcam photos and videos featuring birds, wildlife, farm, and fish and marine life).

If, however, the goal is to create newly developed opportunities for VHAIs, such as through prerecorded videos or synchronous connections, then this would involve a unique set of considerations. In this regard, drawing on our published research developing virtual canine comfort modules to support university students' well-being (Binfet et al., 2022; Tardif-Williams et al., 2023) and the work of other researchers (Dell et al., 2021), we recommend the following evidence-informed best practices. Helping us understand the experiences and perspectives of VHAI participants, we are keen to share their responses to open-ended prompts exploring their thoughts on participating in recent virtual canine comfort sessions. We recognize that not everyone who wishes to create new opportunities for VHAIs will have the same capacity, resources, and funding as university researchers whose job entails work of this nature. What follows is a discussion of the optimal conditions for developing prerecorded videos and offering synchronous sessions. Some of these conditions might be situation specific. Further, it is understood that it might not always be necessary or feasible to implement all these conditions at once. Therefore, we recommend that anyone interested in creating new opportunities for VHAIs draws on the following ideas and suggestions to suit the work they're undertaking.

Personnel Needs

As a starting point, it is wise to consider the personnel needs required to create virtual human-animal connections particularly if one aims to create prerecorded videos or several synchronous sessions. Our work developing virtual canine comfort modules suggests that creating virtual opportunities to engage with animals is an intensive process that often requires input from personnel with expertise across various domains. Thus, a multidisciplinary team is often ideal, and this team could include input from some of the following personnel: researchers, videographers, photographers, animal welfare monitors, experienced dog handlers, monitors to compile/address participants' questions during synchronous sessions, *technology-confident hosts*, video editors, and social media experts. This finding is supported by Dell and colleagues (2021) in their research on transitioning a therapy dog program to an online context during the Covid-19 pandemic. These researchers note that the virtual context is often new for people, and therefore, the staffing and expertise requirements are often greater when designing and producing virtual versus in-person human-animal connections – the process of successfully creating and actualizing VHAIs often requires specific expertise and a larger supporting cast.

Once a goal and method of delivery have been established and a team assembled, additional factors should be considered before creating VHAIs. First, a team must consider if the handlers and animals are well-suited and if they have the necessary skills to feature in VHAIs. Also, the online context might not be equally appealing to all animal handlers. In their research, Dell and colleagues (2021) noted that while they had 35 handlers for their in-person dog program, only 17 dog handlers transitioned to the online context. The handlers who did transition cited their openness to technology and their desire to connect with students and the community as reasons for continuing in the program with their dog.

Handler Training and Preparation

Handler Handbook, Script, and Practice Sessions

It is crucial to carefully consider handler training and preparation when creating virtual human-animal connections. Drawing on our own and others' research, we recommend that teams interested in creating VHAIs should carefully prepare animal handlers for their role in a virtual context, and this might involve a handler training manual, the use of a script (formal or semi-structured), and practice sessions to familiarize handlers and therapy dogs/animals with the room and video equipment (Binfet et al., 2022; Dell et al., 2021; Tardif-Williams et al., 2023).

To begin, handlers will benefit from training and support on the use of technology and their role as handler in a virtual context. They will need to receive guidance in terms of what to do when the filming begins and/or what to say or do when engaging with viewers in a synchronous, real-time context. Toward this goal, we recommend that teams creating VHAIs develop a handler handbook with a script, outline etiquette and expectations (e.g., appropriate attire for sessions, presenting in a friendly and welcoming manner), and detail some key online programming prerequisites (e.g., tips on how to use social media platforms, what platforms are popular, learning the best time to actually post content for maximum views). Handler training will vary depending on the style of the prerecorded video or synchronous sessions that are being created. However, at the very least, handler training should include familiarization with the featured animal(s) (if not already familiar), the filming location or setting in which synchronous VHAIs will take place, and the personnel including the videographer(s) and video equipment.

Handlers should be trained to be present in a calm, welcoming, and inclusive way, to speak in a composed and soothing voice, and to balance their interactions among all virtual group members, including the featured animal. In our research developing virtual canine comfort modules (Tardif-Williams et al., 2023), one participant stated, "I enjoyed how she [handler] spoke with a soothing voice. It calmed me down (Participant 22)." Another participant shared the following, "I thought the study was very professional by the instructor and handler, but also a very safe and calming space to be in. The handler has a great way of making you feel safe (Participant 32)." Also, gleaning insights from research investigating online mental health delivery (Barker &

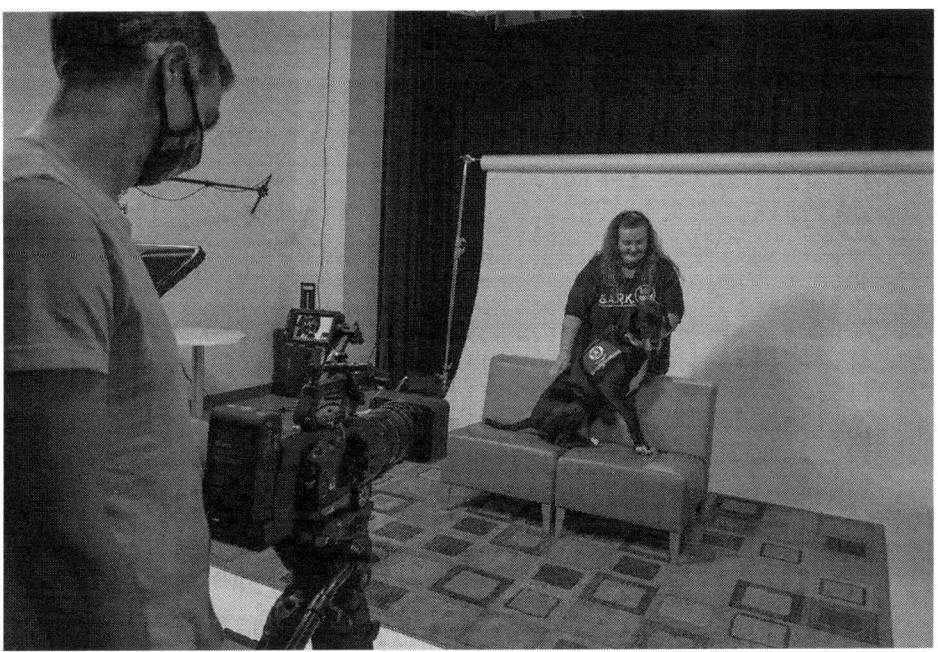

Figure 6.2 Videographer, handler Terina, and her therapy dog Layla from UBC's B.A.R.K. program preparing for a filming session

Source: F. L. L. Green Photography

Barker, 2022; Mallonee et al., 2022), we recommend training handlers to increase their *telepresence*, or to use a clear tone of voice with more verbal affirmations and to be more deliberately overt in their facial expressions and body language. For example, it can be more difficult to interpret the virtual context when people have a limited view of handlers' and animals' gestures, posture, and body movement. Also, *telepresence* can be very helpful for people who have disabilities (e.g., people who have autism or attention deficit hyperactivity disorder) – increasing handler *telepresence* is one way to be more inclusive and sensitive in supporting diverse groups of people. Overall, the role of the handler should not be underestimated. Participants in research conducted by Dell and colleagues (2021) described the handler as a "connection to the dog" (p. 4) – the handler serves as a translator between the client and the dog. Notably, however, the handlers also identified their new role and the virtual setting as very draining. Therefore, we recommend that handlers are prepared in advance of the demands that will be placed on them in their role creating VHAIs and are given breaks as needed during the process of creating and delivering VHAIs. In addition to considering animal welfare throughout the creation of VHAIs, we must consider the welfare of handlers as well as they, too, are key agents making VHAI content possible.

As we noted, one way of supporting handlers is through the use of a formal or semi-structured script to guide handlers on what to say and do during filming or as they facilitate synchronous sessions with animals. To illustrate, in our research developing virtual canine modules, we included a semi-structured script for therapy dog handlers to guide their dialogue with university students during both synchronous (i.e., Zoom or livestream) or asynchronous (i.e., prerecorded) sessions (Tardif-Williams et al., 2023). See Table 6.2 for an example of a script which can be

Table 6.2 Example Script to Guide Handlers During Virtual Human-Animal Interaction Sessions

Handler Script for Virtual Sessions with Animals:
The following script could be used by handlers to guide their dialogue with participants in virtual sessions, whether the sessions take place synchronously (i.e., Zoom or livestream) or asynchronously (i.e., prerecorded) sessions. Welcome to a virtual human-animal session offered by _____ I am an animal handler and my name is _____. My therapy animal(s) participating in today's sessions is/are _____. Let me explain what will happen over the next 5 minutes we're together. First, I will introduce my therapy animal or animal(s) to you and I will ask you some questions to engage you in today's session, similar to what I might ask if you attended an in-person session with a therapy animal(s). Let's begin. Let me introduce you to my therapy animal. His/her name is _____. As you can see, he/she is a _____ (identify type of animal or breed). He/she is _____ years old. *Handler then describes the animal's background including how the animal joined the handler's family, how long the animal has worked as a therapy animal, and some details about the animal's personality and their likes and dislikes.* Now, I'm going to ask you to reflect on how you're doing. We know that being a university student can be a stressful experience. Added to this, you've had to adapt to a virtual or online learning context and that potentially has added stress to your situation. As I ask you these questions, think about your responses and the motivation behind your choices. Also, as you reflect on these questions, I want you to imagine yourself petting _____ (insert animal's name) and getting to know _____ (insert animal's name) even though you may be far away from campus. 1. What brought you to participate in this virtual session with a therapy animal or animal(s)? 2. How are you finding your classes this semester? 3. What activities have you enjoyed participating in recently? Have you joined any clubs or student groups? Have you maintained your hobbies or found new ones? 4. Next, I want you to think about your social support system. Have you made connections to other students? Often, joining the clubs or pursuing hobbies mentioned previously can help you build this network. 5. How are you feeling at this very moment? You're doing something right in accessing this virtual session as virtual sessions like this have been shown to reduce stress. I hope you enjoyed today's session and remember, should you be feeling overwhelmed, you can reach out to your professors, friends, or loved ones for academic and emotional support and you can access the resources available through the Student Services and Wellness Centre.

Source: adapted from Tardif-Williams et al., 2023

easily adapted for use when creating and delivering other types of virtual human-animal connections. The script was designed to reach the following goals: to facilitate introductions among handler, therapy dog and students; to discuss the therapy dog's background, personality, likes, and dislikes; to encourage student reflections on the stressors associated with adapting to the online learning context; and to encourage student visualizations of virtually petting and touching the therapy dog, even if far away from campus. Handler scripts might also include prompts to encourage visualizations of seeing, talking to, or petting animals; enhance mindfulness and relaxation; reflect on stress management techniques; reflect on previous and current experiences with companion animals; and reflect on animal-themed questions or material.

It is also important to note that handlers will need time to learn and practice the script, or they will need to receive coaching on what to say or talk about during VHAIs. One way to do this involves practice sessions for the handler, with and without actual filming and/or synchronous interactions with animals. Last, as part of the handler training, we recommend informing the handler that prerecorded videos will be disseminated to a diverse public audience and available at anytime and anywhere, requiring their informed consent. Teams creating VHAIs will have to consider and negotiate their plans to protect the handlers' and any other participants' confidentiality; this is especially true if teams are filming in the handlers' or participants' personal space, such as in their homes.

Navigating the Animal's Role

In terms of the animals involved in the creation and delivery of virtual human-animal connections, it is of utmost importance that they are screened in advance for suitability and for their own and everyone's safety. Some further considerations include: Is the animal suitable for actualizing VHAIs (e.g., not showing signs of aggression or distress)? Is the animal calm, gentle, and showing a good temperament? Can the animal follow basic instructions, if necessary (e.g., responds to basic obedience commands)? And, can the animal sit for long periods of time and regain self-control after play or excitement, if necessary (Binfet & Hartwig, 2020)? Once it is established that the animal in question is a good fit for creating VHAIs and will assist with the goals of actualizing VHAIs, we recommend that the animal is provided an opportunity to become familiar with the filming location and surroundings in which VHAIs will take place. As with handler training, this might include engaging the animal in several practice sessions with and without actual filming and/or synchronous interactions with people.

As we discussed in Chapters 4 and 5, there are unique animal welfare considerations within virtual contexts. As the field of VHAIs expands, it will be necessary to establish guidelines for safeguarding animal welfare in research and practice. We note several unique considerations when creating VHAIs. For instance, we recommend that animals' suitability for virtual work be assessed early in the process as some animals might become bored or anxious remaining in one spot for lengthy periods during the filming process or while their handler engages with other people. Some animals might not be comfortable with or safe around filming equipment, and still others might not feel comfortable with a filming crew that includes several new people. Therefore, before creating VHAIs, it is important to consider whether the animals will be comfortable with the studio or space in which they will be filmed and what will be done to ensure their comfort if this is not the case. For instance, it might be necessary to reduce the heat in the space as filming lighting creates additional warmth and the space will likely need to be enclosed to reduce noise. Also, if the filming is done in a familiar setting such as the handler's home, then the animal might be more easily distracted and discontent with having unfamiliar visitors carrying large filming equipment into their home. In both familiar and unfamiliar contexts, we recommend that practitioners and researchers interested in creating VHAIs develop a protocol in advance about how to monitor the animals for signs of distress during both the preparation and filming stages. This includes consideration of what action will be taken if an animal voluntarily exits a space and, in this way, does not consent to be involved in a session. As we discussed in Chapter 5, handlers have multiple roles or tasks to perform and will be occupied in their role. Where possible, we recommend assigning a person with the responsibility of monitoring animal welfare throughout the content creation process and terminating a session should an animal show signs of distress.

Technology and Videography

Whether you are creating prerecorded or synchronous VHAIs it is important to begin with high-quality technology and a strong internet connection; this point is also emphasized in studies of

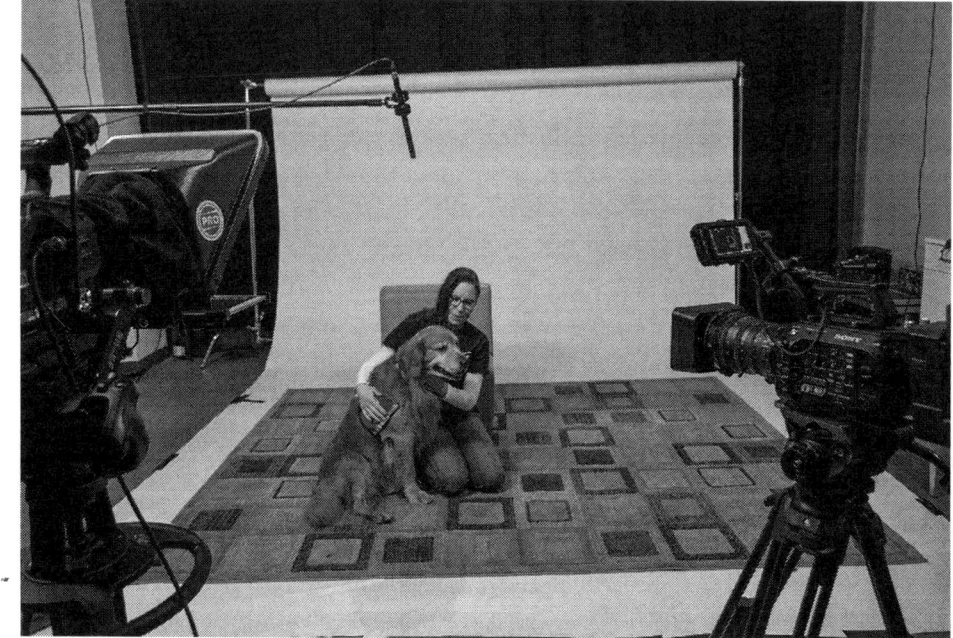

Figure 6.3 Handler Elizabeth and her therapy dog Wrigley from UBC's B.A.R.K. program preparing for a filming session

Source: F. L. L. Green Photography

virtual mental health services more generally (Greiwe, 2022; Mallonee et al., 2022). In a study by Scheck and colleagues (2022) on psychiatric patients' receiving online AAT with dogs during the Covid-19 pandemic, both patients and clinicians reported that the technical difficulties they experienced interfered with their engagement with therapy dog teams.

Moreover, the handlers shared that they found it challenging to sustain the therapy dog's attention throughout the sessions. Findings from our research developing virtual canine comfort modules also support the need for high-quality technology and a strong internet connection (Tardif-Williams et al., 2023). For example, one study participant shared, "It was good. I actually enjoyed talking. Unfortunately, I have a bad internet connection so the session froze on me a few times, so I occasionally missed what the handler said (Participant 10)." Thus, to avoid technical difficulties, we recommend having *technology-confident hosts* available during the creation and delivery of VHAIs. We also recommend having a backup contact plan in case technical difficulties are encountered (e.g., contact by email, text, or phone).

In the case of creating prerecorded VHAIs, it is necessary to first establish the goals and length of videos, the intended audience, and the platform for dissemination (this will inform video format). Next, teams will need to establish some practical details including: Who is going to do the filming? Where will the filming take place? What type of technology will be used to do the filming? Will the filming involve formal or informal VHAIs (e.g., interview or conversational)? Who will edit the video recordings? And who will disseminate the final edited video recordings, and using which platform? In preparation for filming, some consideration regarding the handlers' and animal(s)' appearance is also advised. Handlers and animal(s) should appear looking clean and well-groomed (e.g., hair, clothing), and therapy/working dogs should appear wearing their vests.

Attention to the varied steps or elements of the filming process are important. Polished, professional-looking videos or synchronous VHAIs can be created by using high-quality videography equipment and employing strategies to ensure high-quality digital content. Gleaning insights from research on virtual mental health delivery (Barker & Barker, 2022) and our own research developing canine comfort modules (Binfet et al., 2022), we recommend that teams creating VHAIs focus on setting up the webcam at eye level, dressing in a professional manner, and utilizing a quiet space free of distractions to conduct the sessions. Teams are also encouraged to consult with someone whose hobby is photography, or with a professional photographer (if possible), for guidance about both lighting and camera angles in their efforts to ensure high-quality visuals (e.g., making sure that the camera is at the right angle) and sounds (e.g., blocking out background sounds of voices or wind), which will ensure that the final recordings are polished and professional.

In terms of length, Dell and colleagues (2021) suggest that prerecorded asynchronous videos on social media should be brief, lasting from 1 to 5 minutes, and synchronous meetings should not exceed 20 minutes. Based on our research developing canine comfort modules, we recommend five minutes as a viable length for prerecorded scripted VHAIs. One of our study participants shared, "I think that the length of the video is good . . . near five minutes is a good time for these types of videos. Personally, I would not prefer them to be longer virtually (Participant 347)." Here, we emphasize that there are several stakeholders to consider when planning the duration of VHAIs – the client (to be sure), the handler, and the featured animal. There are also cost implications for creating longer videos, which would require more filming and editing time. Further, longer prerecorded or synchronous scripted VHAIs would require highly engaged

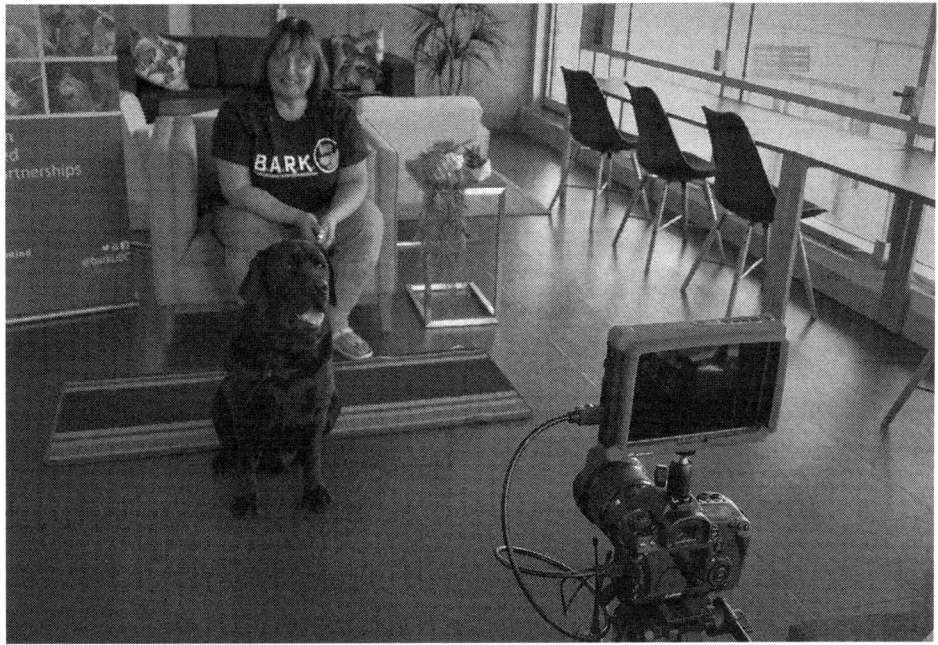

Figure 6.4 Handler Lori and therapy dog MJ from UBC's B.A.R.K. program, centered and looking directly into the camera in preparation for filming

Source: F. L. L. Green Photography

virtual viewers and a focused handler-animal team. Our experience suggests that keeping an animal focused for longer than five minutes is often challenging, and throughout the content creation process, we must aim to safeguard the animal's welfare.

In terms of actual filming, we recommend that teams prepare for multiple takes. The goal is to balance the amount of time needed to capture essential VHAIs, without overextending the duration, which would create strain on the animal(s). Teams should also prepare for contingencies as there will be outtakes and many videos that simply cannot be used (and some that will need to be extensively edited). In our research creating virtual canine comfort modules (Binfet et al., 2022), we planned for two to three takes of each session, with each session lasting approximately an hour. We also planned for return filming visits. Also, post-filming editing is a significant step that can be time-consuming, involving a first round of editing and then subsequent rounds of reviews and edits; this is especially true if teams are aiming to create a video with a specific duration.

Finally, whether they are prerecorded videos or synchronous opportunities, the step of disseminating VHAIs should not be downplayed. Professional videos will reflect positively on the organization, and disseminating content to target audiences is time-consuming. As we discussed in Chapter 4, social media is ever evolving. Some platforms are more popular than others, and different audiences will seek out content on different social media platforms. It is equally important to consider the best time to post prerecorded, or to offer synchronous, VHAIs as some days

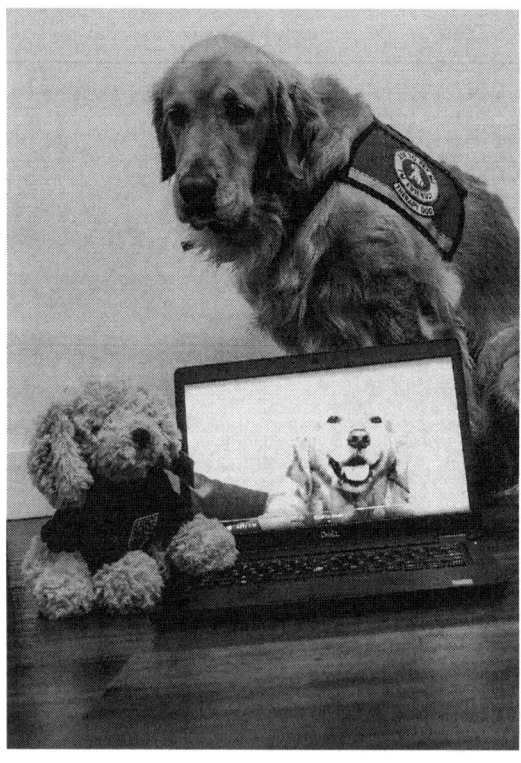

Figure 6.5 Abby, a therapy dog from UBC's B.A.R.K. program, sitting beside a stuffed animal bearing her resemblance and a laptop showing therapy dog Dash on the screen

Source: F. L. L. Green Photography

and times might invite a larger number of virtual viewers. The personnel responsible for dissemination should have a strong understanding of social media, the platforms to use depending on the intended audience, the ideal times to post for the intended audience, and the incentives for viewers to participate. The posts should be appealing and well designed to capture the audience's attention. Depending on the goal for creating VHAIs, teams might also consider sponsoring posts to reach a wider and diverse audience of virtual viewers.

Engaging Virtual Viewers

Turning our attention back to the scenario at the outset of this chapter, Mr. Bhatt knows that his students are highly motivated to interact with dogs and other animals in the classroom, but he wonders if they will be as excited to take part in virtual connections with animals. So far in this book, we have established that some of the documented benefits to humans of in-person interactions with animals (particularly therapy dogs) extend to the virtual context (Binfet et al., 2022; Dell et al., 2021; Scheck et al., 2022; Tardif-Williams et al., 2023; Thelwell, 2015). Moving forward, an essential question to consider is *how* to engage virtual viewers, regardless of whether creating prerecorded or synchronous VHAIs. First, it is important to recognize that some people might have low technological literacy and that it might be necessary to offer *client education*, or brief lessons on how to use certain technological or social media platforms with more frequent check-ins during the delivery of VHAIs. A related point to consider is where people will be accessing VHAIs (e.g., home, library). Although VHAIs are easily accessible, it is important to find a quiet and comfortable space to increase people's participation and engagement. Next, once people feel comfortable using the technology and/or social media platform, the question remains, what specifically draws people to virtual connections with animals and what features sustain people's interest and participation with animals in virtual contexts? Here, as research and practice in the field of VHAIs advances, we recommend several practices to optimize one's reach.

We recommend offering VHAIs using various technology and social media platforms and at various times throughout the weekdays and on weekends; in our recent virtual canine comfort study (Tardif-Williams et al., 2023), our study participants expressed a desire for increased availability of and regular (perhaps weekly) engagement with VHAIs. Still, other participants in our research emphasized the benefit of audience participation in synchronous VHAI group sessions and the use of a moderator to facilitate the process of becoming acquainted with the dog – viewers wanted to learn more about the handler's and dog's lives and their training schedules. It is equally important to consider the length of VHAIs as some viewers will prefer a shorter duration of VHAIs, whereas others will prefer opportunities for longer virtual connections with animals. One participant in our research shared, "If the sessions were longer and we were given more of a chance to develop a deeper relationship with the moderator/the other participants, I think it could have a positive impact (Participant 36)."

This latter quotation suggests that, in addition to connecting virtually with animals, some virtual viewers might seek out and value opportunities to interact socially. Depending on the goal for creating VHAIs or people's preferences, it might be desirable to facilitate or prerecord sessions involving familiar and unfamiliar people. If the goal is to facilitate social connections, then it would make sense to include new and unfamiliar people as part of VHAIs. However, some people might feel anxious participating in VHAIs that include unfamiliar people. This sentiment was nicely articulated by another one of our study participants in the following way, "I feel that being in a group of strangers made the interactions seem awkward and forced and did not necessarily reduce stress. By being in a group of people you are more familiar with, I feel it would allow for more authentic communication and a better experience overall (Participant 81)." Another virtual viewer shared, "I really liked how the groups were small and we were able to feel safe and welcomed (Participant 281)." Yet another participant suggested that VHAIs might be more engaging and exciting if they were able to attend with only a small group of friends. These participants' experiences highlight the importance of attending to social dynamics when creating and delivering VHAIs. For instance, as we discussed in Chapters 1 and 2, besides providing direct social support, animals also act indirectly as social facilitators or social lubricants (Guest et al., 2006; Kruger & Serpell, 2006). Animals often facilitate intimate, one-on-one connections and group interactions, factors theorized to contribute to stress reduction – in this way, animals can also serve a protective function. Moving forward, we contend that these are valuable insights to inform the creation of both prerecorded and synchronous VHAIs.

In terms of how to engage viewers in VHAIs, our own and others' research highlights several key animal-related features to consider. Research by Dell and colleagues (2021) suggests that one way to help people to feel more connected with animals (in this case, dogs) in virtual contexts is to provide more dog-specific information (e.g., dog's favourite toy or birthday). Participants in our research on the impact of virtual canine comfort agreed as highlighted by the following insight: "I think it would be cool to share dog profiles during the session like their name, a cute picture, some backstory, their favourite toy and treat etc. – just an idea (Participant 297)." Another way to engage viewers in VHAIs is to encourage the featured animal to look into the camera and focus their attention on the screen and individual behind the screen as a way to increase people's sense of connection to the animal. Notably, participants in Dell and colleagues' (2021) research described how they felt that the dogs were able to express their love for humans through their facial expressions. This suggestion aligns with the biopsychosocial approach (Gee et al., 2021) and research pointing to the important role of eye gazing in communication between humans and animals. As we discussed in Chapter 1, researchers have identified that mutual eye gazing between dogs and their human companions increases oxytocin levels in both dogs and humans – thus promoting a positive oxytocin loop (Nagasawa et al., 2015; Odendaal & Meintjes, 2003). It is thought that these biological effects may translate to additional positive emotional effects for people (Gee et al., 2021).

Yet another way to engage viewers in VHAIs is to have the featured animals involved in activities (Dell et al., 2021; Tardif-Williams et al., 2023). Research by Scheck and colleagues (2022) on psychiatric patients' experiences of weekly online animal-assisted therapy sessions during the Covid-19 pandemic suggested that interacting virtually with a dog benefited patients' well-being. Importantly, however, although the patients reported that they connected with the therapy dogs, they sometimes felt the connection to be *one-sided* (as compared with in-person sessions), as if they were benefitting from the sessions more than the dogs. Patients also noted that they missed the engagement they felt from being in-person (e.g., petting) and the physical contact with therapy dogs. Our research developing virtual canine comfort modules also supports the benefits of creating more interactive VHAIs (Tardif-Williams et al., 2023). Participants in our research shared the following, "I would have loved if it could have been a little more 'dog' focused. Maybe like watching them do a trick or something (Participant 100)." Another participant shared, "Do one-on-one sessions or post videos of the dogs playing or doing cute things. I think that will be more beneficial for people's well-being. Or make the session more interactive with the dog (Participant 114)."

Similarly, Thomas (2020) argues that conservation education experiences involving virtual (and in-person) zoos and aquariums should include more authentic participatory experiences and free-choice learning opportunities where audiences can discover and learn on their own. We recommend that teams creating VHAIs consider ways to encourage authentic participatory experiences where audiences can engage more directly with the featured animal by requesting that the handler interact with the animal or by speaking one-on-one to the animal (e.g., calling their name). Along these lines, Fernandes et al. (2021) suggest that VHAIs could include participatory and engaging events such as livestreaming animals playing, offering online booking systems for appointments with pets, doing interactive games or yoga with pets, and having giveaways and informative sessions to learn more about animals.

Mindfulness

Here, we draw connections to research on mindfulness and suggest that we can apply key principles of mindfulness (e.g., intention, attention, attitude; Kabat-Zinn, 1994) to enhance the creation and delivery of VHAIs. Mindfulness has been defined as "paying attention in a particular way; on purpose, in the present moment, and non-judgmentally" (Kabat-Zinn, 1994, p. 4). The seven principles of mindfulness are: non-judging, patience, beginner's mind, trust, non-striving, acceptance, and letting go (Kabat-Zinn, 2013). Practicing mindfulness involves a focus on being in the present moment, cultivating kind intention, and being openly aware of your breath, body, thoughts, and inner experiences. Researchers have shown that mindfulness practice can help to improve attention and concentration, relieve stress, reduce symptoms of anxiety and depression, improve sleep (Kabat-Zinn, 2013; Siegel, 2018), and increase self- and other-directed compassion (Neff, 2011).

Animal-themed guided meditations are increasing in popularity as videos can be easily accessed as scripts online or as short videos on YouTube. These guided meditation videos or scripts are designed to encourage mindfulness and guide the participant through breathing exercises to promote relaxation and ease anxiety, increase body awareness, and facilitate visual or tactile imagery involving the featured animal (e.g., visualize that you are gazing into your companion animal's eyes and lovingly stroking their soft fur; visualize walking with your companion animal along a sandy beach on a warm summer day). Using qualitative methodology, Lalonde and colleagues (2020) conducted in-depth interviews with four female university students who attended an on-campus, in-person dog therapy program. Key insights gleaned from these interviews included: *being in-the-moment*, social benefits, variations in coping ability, personalized interactions, and reciprocal interactions. Drawing on these insights, we suggest that one way to engage viewers in VHAIs is to create *mindful moments* (or *being in-the-moment*) and to facilitate guided visual or tactile imagery involving the featured animal. In our own and others' research (Dell et al., 2021; Tardif-Williams et al., 2023), virtual viewers often expressed a desire to *reach across the screen* to touch, see, or communicate with the featured animal. This sentiment is expressed in the following ways by participants in our research on students' experiences of virtual canine comfort modules (Tardif-Williams et al., 2023): "I wish I got to see more of Dash or see the handler petting her to make me imagine petting her myself (Participant 20)," "Maybe let the handler pet the dog? (Participant 324)," and "It makes me think of those videos where you hold eye contact with another person for several minutes and you feel love towards them. Maybe if you did something like that? (Participant 169)."

Further, in another study, researchers examined how the sensory experiences (i.e., sense of *flow* and *social presence*) of individuals who have watched pet videos/livestreams might be associated with their subjective well-being (Zhou et al., 2020). Findings from this study involving 439 young people (aged 21–30 years; 74.55% female) showed that both telepresence (i.e., feeling of *being there*) and social presence (i.e., feeling of *being with others*) had significant positive effects on *flow experience* and that *social presence* had a significant positive impact on subjective well-being. Importantly, this study not only supports the positive effect of online pet watching on subjective well-being, but it also suggests some of the social processes or dynamic nuances undergirding this association.

Therefore, we recommend that practitioners and researchers interested in creating VHAIs facilitate opportunities for virtual viewers to experience *being in-the-moment* or *being there* or *being with others/featured animal(s)*. Toward this goal, we recommend giving virtual viewers the option of asking the handler to touch or pet the featured animal (e.g., Can you pet the horse on his head? Can you rub the dog's tummy?), or to ask the handler questions about the featured animal (e.g., How long have you and your therapy dog been in training? How long have you been raising and caring for rabbits?). Also, it would be wise to consider, whenever possible, giving virtual viewers the option to choose the handler and animal they want to watch/engage with; someone might choose to watch/engage with a handler that reminds them of someone they love or feel comfortable with and/or to watch/engage with a therapy dog that reminds them of their own canine companion.

Each of the previously noted suggestions regarding how to engage virtual viewers aligns with the biopsychosocial approach (Gee et al., 2021), as discussed in Chapter 1, which proposes that people's interactions with dogs (and other animals) may have important impacts on each of the biological, social, and psychological aspects of human health. Our interactions with a dog (or a companion animal) can reduce stress and increase positive affect by reducing cortisol levels (a hormone associated with stress) and releasing oxytocin (a hormone associated with attachment and affiliation – the *love* or *bonding* hormone) (Rault et al., 2017). Also, a social support hypothesis can be applied to explain the physiological and psychological benefits of interacting with companion animals (Fine & Weaver, 2018; O'Haire, 2010). Within the context of VHAIs, the animal and other people interacting with an animal, including an animal handler, can be perceived as a sort of social resource supporting people, bolstering people's ability to cope, and buffering people from the adverse effects of stress.

Developmentally Responsive Virtual Human-Animal Interactions: Engaging Younger Audiences With Diverse Animals

Recall the scenario at the outset of this chapter in which Mr. Bhatt wonders how he might virtually connect his students and his beloved farm animals. While many of the recommendations described previously regarding how to engage virtual viewers will apply equally to a younger audience, we note that engaging a younger audience in VHAIs will also present some unique considerations. To begin, research shows that children often have many different types of companion animals, including dogs, cats, fish, birds, reptiles, and farm and forest animals (e.g., horses, sheep, and chickens), and that children often develop meaningful emotional bonds with these diverse animals (Amiot et al., 2016). Further, in one study, children who participated in a week-long camp-based humane education curriculum involving different animals such as dogs, cats, and farm animals (e.g., donkeys) reported sharing significantly closer relationships and bonds with their home-based companion animals at the end of the week (Tardif-Williams & Bosacki, 2015) and an increased ability to recognize and interpret emotional and mental states (e.g., intentions and desires) in animals (Bosacki & Tardif-Williams, 2019; Tardif-Williams & Bosacki, 2017). These findings suggest that children's experiences with diverse animals at home or within other school- or camp-based contexts are associated with the quality of relationships they share with animals and their ideas about animals' emotional and mental states. We argue in this book that such associations might also be supported through children's virtual connections with animals. Further, virtual contexts hold the promise to connect younger children with diverse animals, animals toward which they express natural curiosity and affinity as per the biophilia hypothesis (Wilson, 1984) introduced in Chapter 1, but that might not be easily included as part of an in-person lesson.

In addition, research indicates that children's understanding about animals and their family-based and cultural experiences with animals are connected to their *belief in animal mind*. *Belief in animal mind* involves attributing mental states to animals, or believing that animals have the ability to think, feel, and experience emotions (Hawkins & Williams, 2016). Importantly, *belief in animal mind* is a sociocognitive ability that develops in early childhood and can influence children's attitudes toward animals and their thoughts about animal welfare (Ellingsen et al., 2010; Hawkins & Williams, 2016). In their research, Hawkins and Williams' (2016) found that children's *belief in animal mind* was positively associated with attachment to companion animals and more positive attitudes and humane behaviour toward animals. In turn, in this same study, the children's acceptance of intentional and unintentional animal cruelty and neglect was negatively associated with their *belief in animal mind* (Hawkins & Williams, 2016).

In another study, Menor-Campos and colleagues (2018) found that Spanish children aged 6–13 years espoused *belief in animal mind*, regardless of the children's age, gender, pet ownership, or the species of the animal. However, the children had more difficulty attributing sentience to animals, particularly animal species which they interacted with less regularly (e.g., cows, frogs, goldfish). Also, children's ability to identify animal emotions increases as a function of the child's age and experiences with companion animals at home (Rocha et al., 2016). Researchers have also shown that companion animals are commonly perceived to have higher cognitive capacities than other animals (Maust-Mohl et al., 2012). Among children, familiarity with certain animals might be associated with a tendency to overestimate mental capacities in these animals (Knight et al., 2004). Further, in a study by Menor-Campos and colleagues (2019), living with a dog or small mammal was associated with Spanish children's (aged 6–13 years) prosocial animal attitudes. Still, other researchers have found that, in the context of pet ownership, the development of child-animal bonds varies as a function of age, with older children (aged 11–14 years) developing bonds more easily with species that are not behaviourally similar to humans (e.g., reptiles, fish) and younger children (aged 6–10 years) showing a preference towards species behaviourally closer to humans (e.g., dogs, cats; Hirschenhauser et al., 2017).

These findings point to the importance of animal-related experiences and education across several contexts (e.g., home, camp) in shaping children's learning and knowledge about diverse animals. Again, we submit that these latter associations might also be supported through children's virtual connections with animals. Clearly, Mr. Bhatt's goal of virtually connecting his students with his beloved farm animals holds the potential to support student learning about animals and is well-aligned with recent efforts in European and North American schools to promote environmental conservation and to encourage children and youth to reconnect with nature and animals (Bekoff, 2014; Crain, 2014). However, it is not always feasible for educators or practitioners to offer younger audiences these types of in-person opportunities to meet a diversity of animals. As such, future research is needed that explores best practices to engage younger children in VHAIs and how children's virtual connections with a diversity of animals including farm animals might shape their learning or understanding of companion, farm, and wild animals and their beliefs about, attitudes toward, and treatment of these animals.

In terms of creating developmentally responsive VHAIs, researchers, educators and practitioners are encouraged to offer opportunities early in the curriculum with younger children to promote the development of knowledge about animals, *belief in animal mind*, and positive relationships with and treatment toward animals. Research clearly outlines the importance of children's family-based, cultural, and educational experiences with diverse animals in shaping children's developing ideas about animals. Drawing on the available research, VHAIs with younger children (aged 6–10 years) could include more familiar animals such as cats and dogs to build on children's preference for animals with whom they have more experience or for species behaviourally closer to humans. Virtual human-animal connections with older children or adolescents (aged 11–14 years) could include a greater range of animals or species that are less behaviourally similar to humans (e.g., reptiles, fish). In addition, as discussed in Chapter 3, virtual human-animal connections might be especially important for younger children who are unable to have a companion animal at home; these children would then reap the learning, social. and well-being benefits of virtually interacting with animal(s).

Assessing the Benefits of Virtual Human-Animal Opportunities on Participants

Looking forward to what is needed in the field of VHAIs, we emphasize the need for both systematic and informal assessments of the impact of virtual connections with animals on diverse participants. More generally, the field of HAIs and AATs continues to be characterized by concerns that research assessing the impact and effectiveness of humans' connections with animals is not adequately rigorous. There are continued calls to develop studies that include control conditions, random assignment of participants to treatment and control conditions, multiple measures, long-term post-intervention or treatment follow-up, and the inclusion of manuals to standardize intervention or treatment procedures (for a discussion, see Herzog, 2015; Kerns et al., 2023).

These same methodological and assessment concerns apply to the burgeoning field of VHAIs. Therefore, moving forward, teams creating and developing VHAIs should be committed to the systematic assessment of the impact of VHAIs on their intended audience. Assessing the impact of VHAIs on participants can be a challenging undertaking and requires teams to carefully revisit their goals for creating and delivering VHAIs. For instance, educators such as Mr. Bhatt featured in this chapter's opening scenario might be keen to assess different aspects of students' learning, reading, social connections, or well-being. Still, other researchers and educators will want to know if virtual connections with animals are associated with more empathic treatment toward animals and increased knowledge about animals' habitats, behaviours, and social needs and welfare, whereas practitioners (and researchers) will be especially interested in assessing the impact of VHAIs on people's social connections and well-being. Some other common assessments in the field of VHAI research include a focus on stress reduction; feelings of loneliness and homesickness; feelings of happiness, social connectedness and belonging; and the development of friendships. Teams will then need to develop an assessment plan in consultation with a researcher with expertise in the broader field of HAIs, and relevant standardized measures will need to be identified. This adds to the complexity of the expertise required to successfully create, actualize, and assess the impact of VHAIs. It merits noting that people who are interested in creating and delivering VHAIs might do so as an adjunct to their regular practice as an educator or counsellor, and therefore, they might struggle with the capacity, funding, and resources to implement formal assessments of the impact of VHAIs.

Assessment of the impact of VHAIs should consider the extent to which people participate, engage, and enjoy their virtual connections with animals. It is essential that VHAIs are designed and delivered in such a way that they sustain people's interest and enjoyment, whether they are students in a classroom, children or youth attending a summer camp program, clients participating in a counselling session, or elderly adults attending an online social event. Consideration should also be given to the complexity of people's virtual experiences with animals. This is in keeping with a focus on principles of equity, diversity, inclusion, and Indigeneity in the creation, actualization, and assessment of VHAIs. For instance, research by Myrick (2015) examined the complexity of emotional reactions associated with viewing online cat-related videos. In this study, viewing online cat-related content was associated with participants' experiences of positive emotions and energizing feelings post-viewing. However, results also showed that when participants watched online cat videos as a means of procrastination, they experienced guilt or a sense of *guilty pleasure,* which can decrease enjoyment and positive emotions post-viewing.

Further, as discussed previously, research with children suggests that pro-animal attitudes and the tendency to attribute sentience to animals are linked to knowledge about and with family-based and cultural experiences with animals (Hawkins & Williams, 2016; Menor-Campos et al., 2018, 2019). There is also evidence that children's ability to identify animal emotions increases significantly as a function of the child's age and experiences with companion animals at home (Rocha et al., 2016). These findings point to the importance of animal-related experiences and education in shaping children's ideas about animals and, possibly, their experiences of VHAIs. Future research is needed that examines if, and for whom and under what conditions, viewing online animal-related content or engaging in VHAIs might be associated with both emotional benefits and drawbacks.

As we discussed in previous chapters, VHAIs hold the potential to reach and support diverse audiences, and researchers and educators could develop specialized curricula in inclusive and sensitive ways to support varied groups of people. Therefore, another key dimension to be considered is the extent to which assessment takes into account aspects of diversity in people's experiences with VHAIs. For instance, specialized assessments could explore the extent to which VHAIs appeal to audiences including, but not limited to, people who have disabilities and people within BIPOC and 2SLGBTQI+ communities. In this way, the assessment of VHAIs can include the experiences of different audiences and can begin to address issues of equity, diversity, inclusion, and Indigeneity.

Last, future research on the impact of VHAIs for participants should consider the animal handlers who play a key role is facilitating well-being benefits in participants. Participants in our research (Tardif-Williams et al., 2023) and in research conducted by Dell and colleagues (2021) stressed how the dog handler also helped to facilitate a sense of community within virtual sessions. To be sure, the role of the animal handler has been largely under-investigated in the field of HAIs more generally (Roma et al., 2021; Rousseau et al., 2020). Future research on the impact of VHAIs for participants could explore handlers' characteristics and skills and how these factors might impact the delivery and impact of VHAIs for participants.

Conclusion

Interest in creating virtual human-animal connections is growing among researchers, educators, school and camp counsellors, and practitioners alike. Building upon the foundational information shared thus far in our book, in this chapter, we challenged readers to consider their goals for creating VHAIs. As promised, we provided readers with recommendations for best practices and offered a checklist supporting and guiding readers in the creation and actualization of VHAIs. We discussed the mechanics of how best to design, structure, and deliver VHAIs, including considerations of handler training and preparation, the use of scripts, and technology and videography. Our discussion also addressed some complexities and key challenges in creating and delivering VHAIs and, importantly, how these might be overcome. Drawing on our own and other's research, we then discussed ways to engage virtual viewers and how the application of principles of mindfulness can enhance the delivery of VHAIs. We concluded with a discussion of the assessment of the benefits of virtual connections with animals on participants. We hope that researchers, educators, and practitioners will be inspired by the exciting possibilities for creating and delivering VHAIs to support learning, social connections, and well-being among a diverse group of people. We now turn to a summary of the book including a glance to the future of VHAIs.

References

Amiot, C., Bastian, B., & Martens, P. (2016). People and companion animals: It takes two to tango. *BioScience*, *66*(7), 552–560.

Barak, A., & Grohol, J. M. (2011). Current and future trends in internet-supported mental health interventions. *Journal of Technology in Human Services*, *29*(3), 155–196. https://doi.org/10.1080/15228835.2011.616939

Barker, G. G., & Barker, E. E. (2022). Online therapy: Lessons learned from the covid-19 health crisis. *British Journal of Guidance & Counselling*, *50*(1), 66–81. https://doi.org/10.1080/03069885.2021.1889462

Bekoff, M. (2014). *Rewilding our hearts: Building pathways of compassion and coexistence*. New World Library.

Binfet, J. T., & Hartwig, E. K. (2020). *Canine-assisted interventions: A comprehensive guide to credentialing therapy dog teams*. Routledge.

Binfet, J. T., Tardif-Williams, C., Draper, Z. A., Green, F. L. L., Singal, A., Rousseau, C. X., & Roma, R. (2022). Virtual canine comfort: A randomized controlled trial of the effects of a canine-assisted intervention supporting undergraduate wellbeing. *Anthrozoös*, *35*(6), 809–832. https://doi.org/10.1080/08927936.2022.2062866

Bosacki, S. L., & Tardif-Williams, C. Y. (2019). Children's mental state talk, empathy and attachments to companion animals. *Psychology of Language & Communication*, *23*(1), 284–301. https://doi.org/10.2478/plc-2019-0013

Crain, W. C. (2014). *The emotional lives of animals and children: Insights from a farm sanctuary*. Turning Stone Press.

Crowley, E. J., Silk, M. J., & Crowley, S. L. (2021). The educational value of virtual ecologies in Red Dead Redemption 2. *People and Nature*, *3*(6), 1229–1243. https://doi.org/10.1002/pan3.10242

Davies, E. B., Morriss, R., & Glazebrook, C. (2014). Computer-delivered and web-based interventions to improve depression, anxiety, and psychological well-being of university students: A systematic review and meta-analysis. *Journal of Medical Internet Research*, *16*(5). https://doi.org/10.2196/jmir.3142

Day, V., McGrath, P. J., & Wojtowicz, M. (2013). Internet-based guided self-help for university students with anxiety, depression and stress: A randomized controlled clinical trial. *Behaviour Research and Therapy*, *51*(7), 344–351. https://doi.org/10.1016/j.brat.2013.03.003

Dell, C., Williamson, L., McKenzie, H., Carey, B., Cruz, M., Gibson, M., & Pavelich, A. (2021). A commentary about lessons learned: Transitioning a therapy dog program online during the covid-19 pandemic. *Animals*, *11*(3), 914. https://doi.org/10.3390/ani11030914

Ein, N., Gervasio, J., Reed, M. J., & Vickers, K. (2022). Effects on wellbeing of exposure to dog videos before a Stressor. *Anthrozoös*, 1–19. https://doi.org/10.1080/08927936.2022.2149925

Ein, N., Reed, M. J., & Vickers, K. (2020). Effect of tranquil and active video representations of an unfamiliar dog on subjective mental states. *Society & Animals*, *30*(4), 445–460. https://doi.org/10.1163/15685306-bja10019

Ein, N., Reed, M. J., & Vickers, K. (2021). The effect of dog videos on subjective and physiological responses to stress. *Anthrozoös*, *35*(3), 463–482. https://doi.org/10.1080/08927936.2021.1999606

Ellingsen, K., Zanella, A. J., Bjerkås, E., & Indrebø, A. (2010). The relationship between empathy, perception of pain and attitudes toward pets among Norwegian dog owners. *Anthrozoös*, *23*(3), 231–243, DOI: 10.2752/175303710X12750451258931

Fernandes, A., Chae, Y. S., & South, C. S. (2021). An exploratory analysis of virtual delivery alternatives for university-based animal assisted activities during COVID-19. *Purdue e-Pubs*. Retrieved October 19, 2022, from https://docs.lib.purdue.edu/paij/vol4/iss1/6

Fine, A. H., & Weaver, S. J. (2018). The human – animal bond and animal-assisted intervention. In M. van den Bosch & W. Bird (Eds.), *Oxford textbook of nature and public health: The role of nature in improving the health of a population, Oxford Textbooks in Public Health* (pp. 132–138). Oxford. https://doi.org/10.1093/med/9780198725916.003.0028

Gee, N. R., Rodriguez, K. E., Fine, A. H., & Trammell, J. P. (2021). Dogs supporting human health and well-being: A biopsychosocial approach. *Frontiers in Veterinary Science, 8*. https://doi.org/10.3389/fvets.2021.630465

Greiwe, J. (2022). Telemedicine lessons learned during the covid-19 pandemic. *Current Allergy and Asthma Reports, 22*(1), 1–5. https://doi.org/10.1007/s11882-022-01026-1

Guest, C. M., Collis, G. M., & McNicholas, J. (2006). Hearing dogs: A longitudinal study of social and psychological effects on deaf and hard-of-hearing recipients. *Journal of Deaf Studies and Deaf Education, 11*(2), 252–261. https://doi.org/10.1093/deafed/enj028

Hawkins, R. D., & Williams, J. M. (2016). Children's beliefs about animal minds (child-BAM): Associations with positive and negative child – animal interactions. *Anthrozoös, 29*(3), 503–519. https://doi.org/10.1080/08927936.2016.1189749

Herzog, H. (2015). The research challenge: Threats to the validity of animal assisted therapy studies and suggestions for improvement. In A. H. Fine (Ed.), *Handbook on animal-assisted therapy: Theoretical foundations and guidelines for practice* (pp. 402–407). Elsevier Academic Press.

Hintz, S., Frazier, P. A., & Meredith, L. (2015). Evaluating an online stress management intervention for college students. *Journal of Counseling Psychology, 62*(2), 137–147. https://doi.org/10.1037/cou0000014

Hirschenhauser, K., Meichel, Y., Schmalzer, S., & Beetz, A. M. (2017). Children love their pets: Do relationships between children and pets co-vary with taxonomic order, gender, and age? *Anthrozoös, 30*(3), 441–456. https://doi.org/10.1080/08927936.2017.1357882

Kabat-Zinn, J. (1994). *Wherever you go there you are: Mindfulness meditation in everyday life.* Hyperion.

Kabat-Zinn, J. (2013). *Full catastrophe living (Revised Edition): Using the wisdom of your body and mind to face stress, pain, and illness.* Bantam Books.

Kerns, K. A., Dulmen, M. H., Kochendorfer, L. B., Obeldobel, C. A., Gastelle, M., & Horrowitz, A. (2023). Assessing children's relationships with pet dogs: A multi-method approach. *Social Development, 32*(1), 98–116. https://doi.org/10.1111/sode.12622

Knight, S., Vrij, A., Cherryman, J., & Nunkoosing, K. (2004). Attitudes towards animal use and belief in animal mind. *Anthrozoös, 17*(1), 43–62. https://doi.org/10.2752/089279304786991945

Kogan, L. R., Hellyer, P. W., Clapp, T. R., Suchman, E., McLean, J., & Schoenfeld-Tacher, R. (2018). Use of short animal-themed videos to enhance veterinary students' mood, attention, and understanding of pharmacology lectures. *Journal of Veterinary Medical Education, 45*(2), 188–194. https://doi.org/10.3138/jvme.1016-162r

Kruger, K. A., & Serpell, J. A. (2006). Animal-assisted interventions in mental health: Definitions and theoretical foundations. In A. H. Fine (Ed.), *Handbook on animal-assisted therapy: Theoretical foundations and guidelines for practice* (pp. 21–38). Academic Press. https://doi.org/10.1016/b978-0-12-381453-1.10003-0

Lalonde, R., Dell, C., & Claypool, T. (2020). PAWS your stress: The student experience of therapy dog programming. *Canadian Journal for New Scholars in Education, 11*(2), 78–90.

Mallonee, J., Gergerich, E., Gherardi, S., & Allbright, J. (2022). The impact of covid-19 on social work mental health services in the United States: Lessons from the early days of a global pandemic. *Social Work in Mental Health, 20*(5), 497–516. https://doi.org/10.1080/15332985.2022.2028272

Maust-Mohl, M., Fraser, J., & Morrison, R. (2012). Wild minds: What people think about animal thinking. *Anthrozoös, 25*(2), 133–147. https://doi.org/10.2752/175303712X13316289505224

Menor-Campos, D. J., Hawkins, R., & Williams, J. (2018). Belief in animal mind among Spanish primary school children. *Anthrozoös, 31*(5), 599–614. doi:10.1080/08927936.2018.1505340

Menor-Campos, D. J., Hawkins, R., & Williams, J. (2019). Attitudes towards animals among Spanish primary school children. *Anthrozoös, 32*(6), 797–812.

Myrick, J. G. (2015). Emotion regulation, procrastination, and watching cat videos online: Who watches internet cats, why, and to what effect? *Computers in Human Behavior, 52,* 168–176. https://doi. org/10.1016/j.chb.2015.06.001

Nagasawa, M., Mitsui, S., En, S., Ohtani, N., Ohta, M., Sakuma, Y., Onaka, T., Mogi, K., & Kikusui, T. (2015). Oxytocin-gaze positive loop and the coevolution of human-dog bonds. *Science, 348*(6232), 333–336. https://doi.org/10.1126/science.1261022

Neff, K. (2011). *Self-compassion: The proven power of being kind to yourself.* Harper Collins.

Odendaal, J. S. J., & Meintjes, R. A. (2003). Neurophysiological correlates of affiliative behaviour between humans and dogs. *The Veterinary Journal, 165*(3), 296–301. https://doi.org/10.1016/ s1090-0233(02)00237-x

O'Haire, M. (2010). Companion animals and human health: Benefits, challenges, and the road ahead. *Journal of Veterinary Behavior, 5*(5), 226–234. https://doi.org/10.1016/j.jveb.2010.02.002

Rault, J.-L., van den Munkhof, M., & Buisman-Pijlman, F. T. (2017). Oxytocin as an indicator of psychological and social well-being in domesticated animals: A critical review. *Frontiers in Psychology, 8.* https://doi.org/10.3389/fpsyg.2017.01521

Rocha, S., Gaspar, A., & Esteves, F. (2016). Developing children's ability to recognize animal emotions – What does it take? A study at the zoo. *Human-Animal Interaction Bulletin, 4*(2), 59–79.

Roma, R. P. S., Tardif-Williams, C. Y., Moore, S. A., & Bosacki, S. L. (2021). A transdisciplinary perspective on dog-handler client interactions in animal assisted activities for children, youth, and young adults. *Human-Animal Interaction Bulletin, 9*(2). 62–91.

Rousseau, C. X., Binfet, J. T., Green, F. L. L., Tardif-Williams, C., Draper, Z., & Maynard, A. (2020). Up the leash: An investigation of handler well-being and perceptions of volunteering in canine-assisted interventions. *Pet Behavior Science, 10,* 15–35. https://doi.org/10.2107/pbs.vi10.12598I

Scheck, H., Williamson, L., & Dell, C. A. (2022). Understanding psychiatric patients' experience of virtual animal-assisted therapy sessions during the COVID-19 pandemic. *People and Animals: The International Journal of Research and Practice, 5*(1). https://docs.lib.purdue.edu/paij/vol5/iss1/6

Siegel, D. (2018). *Aware: The science and practice of presence – the groundbreaking meditation practice.* Tarcherperigee.

Tardif-Williams, C. Y., Binfet, J. T., Green, F. L. L., Roma, R., Akshat, S., Rousseau, C. X., & Godard, R. J. (2023). When therapy dogs provide virtual comfort: Exploring university students' insights and perspectives. *People and Animals: The International Journal of Research and Practice, 6*(1), 1–17. https://docs. lib.purdue.edu/paij/vol6/iss1/5

Tardif-Williams, C. Y., & Bosacki, S. (2015). Evaluating the impact of a humane education summer camp program on school-aged children's relationships with companion animals. *Anthrozoös, 28*(4), 587–600.

Tardif-Williams, C. Y., & Bosacki, S. L. (2017). Gender and age differences in children's perceptions of self-companion animal interactions expressed through drawings. *Society and Animals, 25,* 77–97.

Thelwell, E. L. R. (2015). Paws for thought: A controlled study investigating the benefits of interacting with a house-trained dog on university students mood and anxiety. *Animals, 9*(10), 846. https://doi. org/10.3390/ani9100846

Thomas, S. (2020). Social change for conservation – the world zoo and aquarium conservation education strategy. *International Zoo Educators Association.* Retrieved October 19, 2022, from https://izea.net/ the-waza-education-strategy/

Wilson, E. O. (1984). *Biophilia.* Harvard University Press.

Zhou, Z., Yin, D., & Gao, Q. (2020). Sense of presence and subjective well-being in online pet watching: The moderation role of loneliness and perceived stress. *International Journal of Environmental Research and Public Health, 17*(23), 9093. https://doi.org/10.3390/ijerph17239093

7 Conclusion and Future Directions

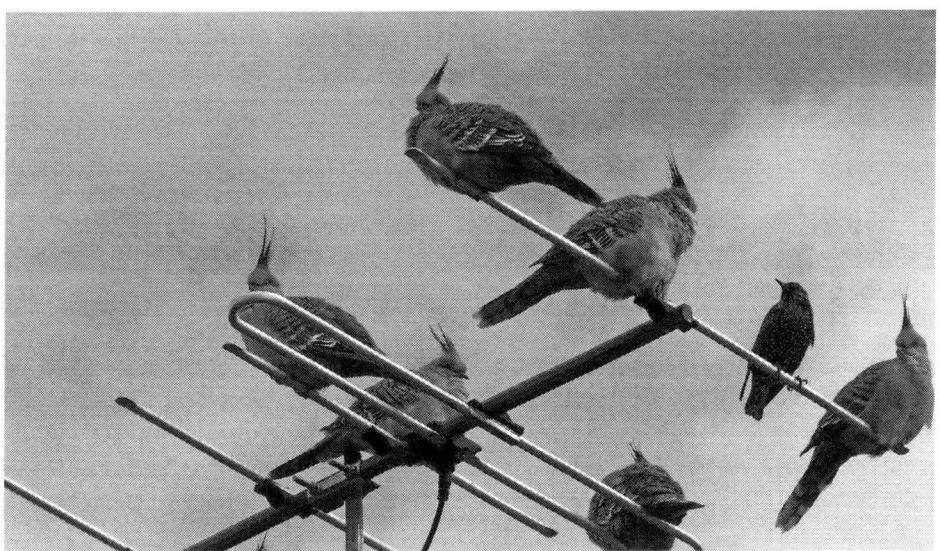

Figure 7.1 Birds pass commentary on technology by roosting on old antennae
Source: Pixabay

Scenario

Dogs watching television?

After moving in together, and much to the chagrin of their parents, millennials Liam and Lucy purchased a French bulldog they named Brian. Brian quickly became a valued family member, and many of Liam and Lucy's weekly activities revolved around outings with Brian, organizing playdates with other dogs in the neighborhood, taking him to the local pub, and bringing him to the weekly Sunday night family dinner. At a recent dinner, Liam asked for the television to be turned on so that Brian could watch a show on DogTV's Youtube channel while the family ate. Frustrated by this request, Liam's father said: "This is too much. Dogs don't need to be entertained by TV shows! You're taking this pet parenting too far. He eats organic food, you watch his every move on multiple nanny cams stationed throughout your apartment, he sleeps in your bed, and he's constantly dressed in new outfits. Listen, there will be no TV for Brian tonight. When you get home, throw a ball for him. That's the entertainment he needs."

DOI: 10.4324/9781003327868-7

Questions for Reflection

1. Are there generational differences in how humans and animals interact?
2. What are the entertainment needs of companion animals? Do animals enjoy watching television?
3. How has technology shifted how humans interact with animals and how humans care for pets?
4. What are the similarities and differences in child- and pet-rearing practices?

Our overarching goal in writing this book was to extend the discussion of human-animal interactions by exploring and examining the role of technology in facilitating VHAIs. In our opening scenario, we see an example of a young couple embracing technology to the extent they provide opportunities for their dog to watch species-specific television programming. Tension over pet parenting beliefs is evident when a dog's television viewing clashes with a family dinner. As convenient as technology can render our lives, it can also introduce complexities.

The aim of this last chapter is to review key concepts introduced in each of the chapters comprising this book and synthesize these concepts as we identify future directions informing VHAIs. We'll begin by revisiting the themes showcased within each chapter's opening scenario – scenarios that challenged our thinking around how we interact with animals and the role that technology plays in our interactions. Next, we'll revisit key arguments in favor of VHAIs as well as briefly review some of the cutting-edge research attesting to the benefits of VHAIs. Last, we'll cast an eye to the future and identify areas for further exploration and discovery.

Synthesizing the Themes Found Within Each Chapter's Opening Scenario

In Chapter 1, we saw a single parent struggling to respond to meet the needs of her children – one allergic to pets and the other desperately wanting a kitten. Here we saw a mother wondering if a *virtual pet* might be the solution. In Chapter 2, we saw a young college student with compromised mental health seek help by trying to attend a popular on-campus canine-assisted stress-reduction program. He's dismayed at the long line to attend and wonders why he can't just spend time with therapy dogs virtually. After all, he lives most of his life within a virtual context, shopping, socializing with his peers, and even attending classes virtually. The scenario in Chapter 3 showcased how technology enriched the life of a senior citizen in a care facility with a fondness for watching wild birds at feeders. Watching livestream video of birds enriched the quality of this senior's life and served to connect her to her daughter. In Chapter 4, we saw how technology posed a parenting challenge for a family when a young son begs his parents to let him use social media to create an Instagram account for their pets. Arguing it would be a harmless way to celebrate the lives of their pets and that he'd only share the account with friends leaves the parents wondering if this is in their child's best interest. Does pet-based social media alter how we interact with companion animals? Moving beyond domestic animals to consider our interactions with wildlife, the scenario in Chapter 5 showcased how technology in the form of a trail cam compromised the well-being of wildlife in a busy urban park. The trail cam viewers, eager to engage with wildlife, suggested leaving food to entice wildlife to spend more time in front of the camera. Here we saw an example of how technology and animal welfare collided. Whereas the scenario in Chapter 5 compromised animal welfare, the scenario in Chapter 6 illustrated the potential of technology to enrich the curriculum for elementary students as well as their knowledge of varied animals – animals inaccessible to them for in-person interactions because of allergies and other obstacles. The teacher here was considering leveraging technology to enhance students' virtual interactions with animals. Our last scenario presented here in this chapter, illustrates how tensions can arise from the use of technology – especially when intergenerational views, family dynamics, and beliefs around the care of a companion animal inform our understanding of human-animal interactions.

Across these scenarios, we saw a variety of people, animals, and contexts brought together or face challenges as a result of technology. Certainly, one theme evident in many of the scenarios was the issue of welfare – welfare of both animals and humans. Illustrations of how technology holds potential to compromise welfare within the context of VHAIs was evident in Chapter 4 when a preadolescent child asks his parents for permission to create a social media account to share photos of the family's pets. On the one hand, we might consider this child's eagerness to celebrate his connections with his companion animals as a reflection of healthy child-pet bonding. On the other hand, parents may be leery to grant permission in light of the safety and mental health concerns arising from children engaging with social media. The welfare of wildlife was also positioned as front and center in Chapter 5's scenario that described a misguided attempt to entice wildlife to spend time in front of an urban trail cam so that YouTube viewers could watch animals up close. In this scenario, technology would be considered one agent or element compromising the welfare of animals. Technology, in this case, served to encourage unnatural behaviours by baiting wildlife with a pizza left in an urban forest. Rather, technology here served as the catalyst to introduce harm and compromise welfare. Extending the implications of technology further, the role it played here was to misinform the public about how humans should engage with wildlife.

It is our hope that each chapter's scenario will initiate discussion and reflection and challenge the thinking of readers around the role of technology in enriching, facilitating, or compromising human-animal interactions.

The Advantages of Virtual Human-Animal Interactions

Throughout this book, we strove to provide evidence-based information and guidelines to assist practitioners and researchers who are interested in creating their own virtual opportunities for humans to interact with animals. Examined next are several of the distinct advantages offered by VHAIs.

The Creation of Virtual Human-Animal Interaction Content Can Be Low-Cost and Safeguard Animal Welfare

As illustrated in Chapter 3 that showcased asynchronous and synchronous opportunities for humans to engage with VHAI content, the creation of virtual content showcasing HAI may be done by program personnel, handlers themselves, or by members of the public. Program personnel, as we saw with the reporting of findings from the randomized controlled trial assessing virtual interactions with therapy dogs by Binfet et al. (2022b), can be created by hiring a videographer and filming sessions within a studio. Where funding and resources permit, this is one approach that may be organized and overseen by HAI program personnel. It offers a distinct advantage in that it provides opportunities for program personnel to evaluate the content being created all the while reducing the burden of responsibility borne when handlers themselves create content.

A more typical pathway by which VHAI content is likely to be created is when handlers film themselves interacting with their therapy animal from the comfort and confines of their own home. An illustration of this was found in innovative research by Dell and colleagues (2021) reviewed in Chapter 3. Dell and colleagues (2021) outlined the complexities involved in transitioning an in-person program to a virtual context requiring handlers to create virtual content themselves. As we argued, handlers in this role have split responsibilities, and their attention must be distributed across managing their animal, managing technology, and responding to viewer requests and needs. In short, handlers creating virtual content themselves is no small undertaking.

Last, an increasingly popular pathway through which VHAI content may be created arises from efforts from the public to showcase digital content celebrating varied aspects of HAIs. Chapter 4 illustrated the breadth of options available to members of the public using different social media platforms to create HAI content. This might include digital content ranging from instructional videos illustrating how to train a horse to load into a trailer for transport, to how to deter squirrels from feasting at wild bird feeders, to how to assess the disposition of a shelter dog. Of course, when the public creates content, this will inevitably result in content of differing quality, and one risk is that the participation of animals is manipulated or coerced in the process of creating content. That is, that animal welfare might be compromised so that virtual content could be created. Such might be the case when food is used to lure or coax animals into engaging in unnatural behaviours or entering unfamiliar contexts (e.g., filming raccoons entering one's kitchen through a dog door to eat alongside the household cat).

Certainly, when VHAI content is created by handlers themselves or by members of the public using their own technology, the cost of creating this content is reduced. This is perhaps why we see such a plethora of VHAI content – it can be created easily using one's own phone within the context in which the human and animal are accustomed to interacting. Added to this, when handlers themselves create HAI content within the context of their home environment, we see animals experiencing less distress than is potentially the case when animals participate in HAIs in the client's environment (e.g., when therapy dogs visit hospitals). The animals are accustomed to and can easily settle when filmed at home whereas adapting to new environments and interacting in-person with one or more clients hold potential to be stress-inducing.

Virtual Human-Animal Interactions Offer Choice and Variety

As illustrated throughout this book, VHAIs may vary considerably in the content they showcase, their presentation format, and their mode of presentation. Although research to date on VHAIs has focused uniquely on examining therapy dogs (e.g., Binfet et al., 2022b; Dell et al., 2021; Scheck et al., 2022; Steel, 2023; Tardif-Williams et al., 2023), informal VHAIs found via social media vary tremendously. This is largely because this virtual content is created and shared by the public and reflects the public's broad and varied interests in animals. We might see trail cams capturing wildlife, livestream videos of wild bird feeders, homemade instructional videos illustrating how to clean an aquarium, or formally organized virtual AAI sessions with a dog handler and therapy dog. Just how this format is made accessible to viewers also varies and two common pathways through which we see this content shared is via asynchronous and synchronous formats. Asynchronously, we typically see prerecorded video content uploaded to various digital platforms for broad distribution (e.g., YouTube) whereas the synchronous streaming of digital HAI content occurs in real-time and may provide opportunities for viewers to virtually interact with the animal or animal-handler team. Illustrations of this might include a viewer who poses a question in a Zoom chat to ask about an animal or a viewer who is able to switch to a different camera angle when watching video of an osprey feeding her young.

Last, asynchronous VHAI content may be used in tandem with synchronous content to augment the viewer's experience. Extending the example of the nest camera to capture an osprey feeding their young, viewers could watch livestream video of the nest cam and subsequently consult archived video footage illustrating various stages of the incubation and hatching process of young chicks. In this regard, the viewer has autonomy to access VHAI content tailored to their interests and suiting their needs. Illustrating the flexibility of VHAIs further, we might see their use combined with in-person HAIs. For example, a college student could attend an on-campus in-person canine-assisted stress-reduction program and later that same week and from the comfort of his dorm access an archived virtual AAI of the very same dog who participated in their in-person session earlier that week.

Virtual Human-Animal Interactions Facilitate Access for Disenfranchised or Marginalized Viewers

A distinct advantage of VHAIs is that they provide access and opportunity for viewers who, for a variety of reasons, cannot or are unlikely to access in-person sessions. Such reasons might include: (1) viewers who are in geographically remote locations where opportunities to interact with animals is limited. This might include individuals who live outside of urban centres known to have in-person HAI programs in operation; (2) viewers who have allergies or phobias that make attending in-person sessions impossible or challenging; and (3) viewers who are reluctant to seek other forms of support to bolster their well-being. To this latter point, VHAIs can support individuals who may be *hard to reach*. This might include people who are unaccustomed to accessing formal resources or who are distrustful of traditional sources of mental health support.

In Chapter 2, we reviewed research by Bennet and Woodman (2019) extolling an equine therapy program designed to support Indigenous clients, and we saw how a HAI program could be tailored to reflect cultural knowledge, practice, and ways of knowing. The appeal of VHAIs can be enhanced by customizing the intervention to reflect both content valued by the viewers and through the use of an approach that is aligned with principles and practices valued by viewers. For example, as storytelling and the wisdom of elders is deeply valued within Indigenous communities, a VHAI comprised of an elder sharing historical stories of the role of animals within Indigenous culture or facilitating a session that allows the elder to share wisdom around how to respect animals within Indigenous communities and beyond might enhance the appeal of VHAIs and, in turn, serve to expand the reach to viewers who might not otherwise find the content or approach enticing.

Virtual Human-Animal Interactions May Be Accessed When Needed, Repeatedly Accessed, and Accessed in the Format Desired by the Viewer

VHAI content can be accessed by the viewer at the time they feel they need the support offered by VHAIs. That is, traditional, in-person sessions are subject to scheduling reliant upon a number of factors including the availability of human-animal teams, space allocations allowing gatherings, and issues of demand surpassing access. As we argued in Chapter 5 in our discussion of animal welfare considerations, in-person AAIs are a complicated affair to organize given the many stakeholders at play. VHAIs sidestep these complexities and may be accessed at a time convenient to the viewer and, if VHAI content is offered asynchronously, may be repeatedly viewed. In this regard, VHAI offers a source of support that is especially low-barrier, convenient, and accessible.

Virtual Human-Animal Interactions Help Reduce the Burden on Formal Mental Health Resources

In Chapter 3, we positioned AAIs as "a complimentary therapeutic approach – not intended to stand on their own as a comprehensive treatment but rather to offer support to clients in addition to other available services (Marcus, 2013; Nepps et al., 2014; Nimer & Lundahl, 2007;

Rossetti & King, 2010)" (Binfet et al., 2022b, p. 4). This interpretation is buoyed by the interpretation of canine-assisted on-campus visitation programs by Pendry and colleagues (2021), who argue that such programs may be especially appealing to individuals who eschew other, more traditional or formal, avenues of seeking help and support. Thus, AAIs, though not intended to stand on their own as a formal mental health intervention, might appeal to individuals who are unlikely to make use of other resources to support their well-being. In this regard, and certainly in regard to VHAIs, though not a comprehensive solution, VHAIs may serve as an appealing, accessible, and temporary source of support accessed at a time when no other resources are available or willing to be accessed.

We, thus, position virtual AAIs and especially VHAIs as one possible well-being resource that people can access that might provide temporary support, and this support may, in turn, render these individuals to be more receptive to, and possibly seek out, more formal sources of support.

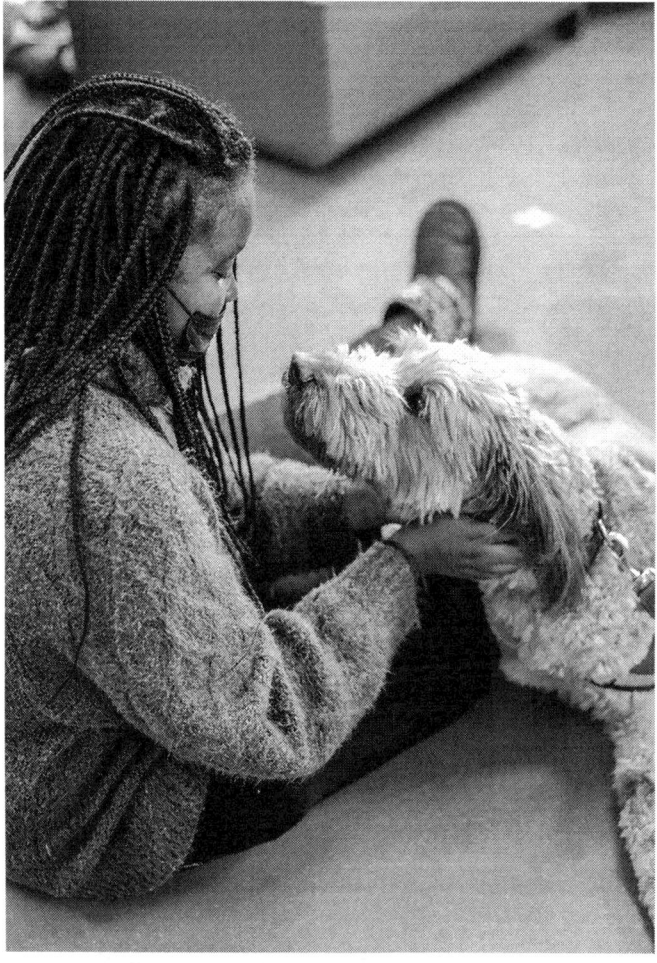

Figure 7.2 A college student interacts with therapy dog Ginny to reduce her stress

Source: F. L. L. Green Photography

As the demand for mental health services rises and in light of current support systems having insufficient capacity to meet this demand, adjunct forms of support such as VHAIs play a particularly valuable role in the mental health landscape. VHAIs hold potential: (1) to offer a gentle, nonthreatening way for individuals to reduce their stress and increase their perception of support; (2) to facilitate individuals seeking additional, more targeted, and formal mental health support; and (3) to provide accessible support to individuals living in underserved communities where options for in-person support are minimal.

The Challenges of Virtual Human-Animal Interactions

Having provided arguments in favor of the use of VHAIs, we now turn to a discussion of the challenges associated with creating and delivering VHAIs.

Recognizing the Shifting Role of the Handler

The role of handlers in VHAIs, especially when creating AAI content for a virtual context, requires both technological proficiency and the managing of multiple stakeholders including their therapy animal and the needs of clients. Handlers, whether they are creating asynchronous content of themselves interacting with their animal or whether they are participating in synchronous sessions in which they interact with their animal, must negotiate and navigate the needs of their animal at the same time as responding to the needs and requests of viewers. As we've argued throughout this book and as has been identified by other researchers, the role of the handler within a virtual context can be a demanding and complicated affair. When compared to an in-person session where the client is able to physically interact with an animal, in a virtual context there is more onus on the handler to keep conversations afloat and to engage the client(s). Handlers may be supported by using a script however the behaviour of their therapy animal as well as questions from viewers must still be managed or addressed.

A second challenge for handlers lies in the possible isolation they experience working in a virtual context. The experiences and motivation of handlers who participate in HAIs remains understudied. Additional research is needed that examines the role of handlers, their experience within HAIs, and their motivation to volunteer. From the scant empirical work exploring who volunteers as a handler in HAIs and their motivation to do so, we know that handlers, certainly within canine-assisted interventions or visitation programs, tend to be middle-aged and female. In a study by Rousseau et al. (2020), 60 volunteer dog handlers in an on-campus stress-reduction program were queried as to why they volunteered with their dog to support student well-being and what they perceived to be the benefits of doing so. In addition to wanting to share their dog with students, handlers identified overwhelmingly that they were motivated to volunteer because of the social enjoyment and benefits they derived. Opportunities to socialize are reduced within a virtual context, and this might pose a threat to recruiting handlers for participation in uniquely virtual sessions.

Potentially Less Robust Effects Than In-Person Animal-Assisted Interventions

We acknowledge that, to date, there is a dearth of research assessing the effects of VHAIs; however, findings from recently published research suggest that the effects of VHAIs on bolstering human well-being are less robust than those elicited from in-person sessions (see Binfet et al., 2022a). In light of the recent evidence indicating that touch (e.g., petting a therapy dog) is a key element contributing to well-being outcomes in humans participating in in-person AAIs (Binfet et al., 2022a), we acknowledge that, though effective, the engagement of virtual clients and their experience in virtual sessions remains distinctly different from clients participating in in-person sessions. This interpretation of virtual canine-assisted interventions was echoed by participants in recent qualitative work exploring undergraduate students' perceptions of spending time virtually with therapy dogs (Tardif-Williams et al., 2023). Students lamented missing the opportunity to have in-person interactions but conceded that the virtual option was better than no option.

As we've argued throughout this chapter and much of the book, VHAIs provide a valuable resource to clients who are geographically isolated, where there may be a distinct lack of well-being resources, or for clients who might not otherwise make use of resources to support their well-being. As we discussed in Chapters 3 and 6, participants in VHAI studies shared how they missed the engagement they felt from being in-person (e.g., petting, giving treats) and the physical contact with therapy dogs. Still, as acknowledged by participants in our own research (Tardif-Williams et al., 2023) and echoed by participants in Scheck et al.'s (2022) research, participants were grateful to access VHAIs especially during the Covid-19 pandemic. Next, we explore areas in which VHAIs might be further researched.

Casting an Eye to the Future of Virtual Human-Animal Interactions

Technology is ever changing, and this represents exciting opportunities for applied and empirical forays into VHAIs. As technological advances are made, opportunities for different iterations of VHAIs are possible. Figure 7.3 depicts a typical on-campus session that brings together unfamiliar students and a dog-handler team. As is typical, the handler will facilitate students getting to know one another, but the role of dogs as social catalysts within a virtual context remains

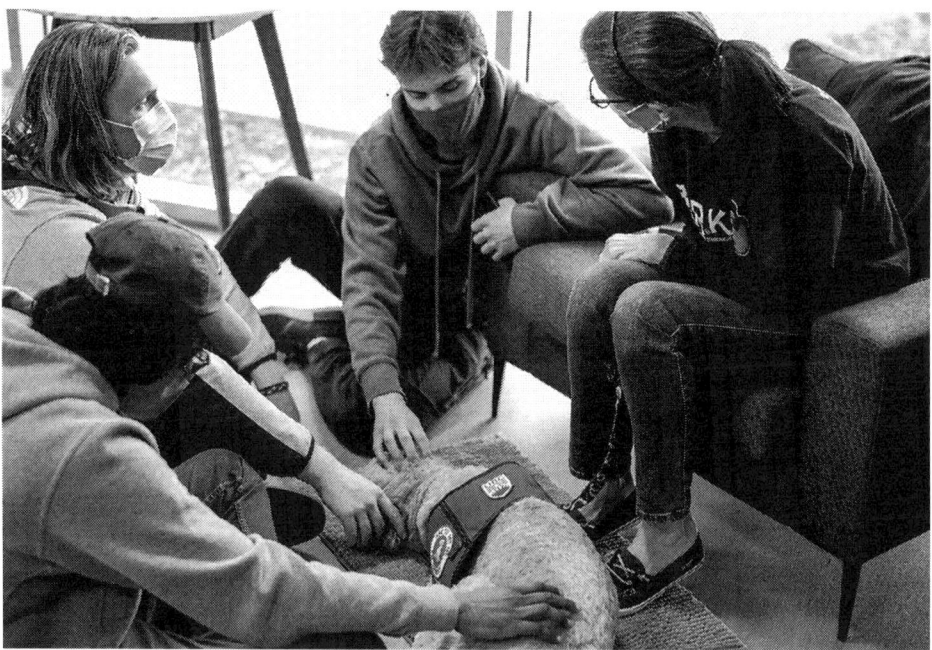

Figure 7.3 Therapy dog Chloe facilitating social interactions as part of an animal-assisted intervention

Source: F. L. L. Green Photography

understudied. In Chapter 3, we reviewed the role of dogs in AAIs connecting people to one another. Might therapy animals working in virtual contexts elicit similar socialization effects? Are some animals particularly well-suited to working in a virtual context? What is the impact of individual versus group-administered VHAIs? Do multiple virtual sessions impact well-being outcomes to a greater extent than single, abbreviated sessions? These, among other questions, are explored next as we look to the future of research in VHAIs.

One area requiring empirical investigation includes how species variability impacts virtual client engagement and motivation. As we recognize in our book, there is a preponderance of programs and research in which dogs are positioned as the therapeutic partner (horses to a lesser extent). VHAIs provide opportunities for other species to participate in sessions and this includes cats – a species who may potentially thrive in virtual sessions given they are able to work in the comfort and security of their familiar home environment. As we discussed in Chapter 6, additional research assessing the effects of VHAIs with different species will help us understand the effects of virtual engagement with different animals (i.e., farm and wild) on dimensions of learning and human well-being from early childhood to adulthood. Akin to cats participating in VHAIs, a virtual format provides opportunities for farm animals to participate in sessions, thereby providing unique opportunities for clients from urban environments, where farm animals are infrequently encountered, to become engaged.

Related to this idea, what are the experiences, implications, and effects of in-person versus virtual participation on animal welfare? In Chapter 5, we acknowledged that virtual AAIs hold potential to reduce stress on animals having to adjust to new environments and to interactions with clients typical of in-person AAIs. We posited (as have Ein et al., 2022 in their recent research on the effects of dog videos on viewer well-being) that participation in virtual AAIs is likely to be less stressful on the animal. Thus, future research examining the effects of in-person versus virtual participation on animal welfare is another area of research requiring exploration.

Research exploring the skills of handlers volunteering in VHAIs is needed. We might ask: "Do in-person skills transfer to virtual contexts?" and "What strategies can handlers employ to engage virtual viewers?" As well, research understanding the experience of handlers volunteering in VHAIs is needed to fully understand the role of these key stakeholders. As handlers are often motivated to participate in AAIs because of the social benefits derived (Rousseau et al., 2020), are handlers' social needs met when volunteering within a virtual context?

Another area of research requiring additional empirical attention is the role that asynchronous and synchronous sessions play in affecting client well-being. Rigorous research designs that assign varied clients to repeated sessions to determine how the technological pathway of access impacts outcomes is needed. Relatedly, how does the content of VHAIs itself impact client engagement and well-being outcomes? Do clients respond in different ways to varied VHAI content? As we discussed in Chapter 4, there is emerging research by Ein et al. (2022) examining the activity levels of dogs within a virtual AAI as a factor impacting viewer well-being. Empirical work investigating varied aspects of the animal's role within the virtual content used as part of the intervention is required. Last, just as researchers have examined the effects of varying AAI durations (e.g., Barker et al., 2016; Binfet et al., 2018) including the use of abbreviated in-person interventions, this remains an area of future study to understand how the duration of participation in virtual AAI content impacts outcome variables. There is nascent research attesting to the efficacy of a 5-minute virtual canine-assisted intervention (Binfet et al., 2022b; Tardif-Williams et al., 2023) yet additional research is required to understand if longer virtual sessions and the use of repeated sessions over time produce stronger effects.

Another area of empirical inquiry worthy of exploration involves the promise of VHAIs to reconnect people with nature. This includes understanding lessons learned from nature, examples of rewilding formerly captive animals, and sensitizing people's hearts toward nature and animals through illustrations of virtual human-animal connections (Bekoff, 2014). As we discussed in Chapter 1, people's increased use of technology is often juxtaposed with their tendency to be less engaged with the natural world and animals. Some scholars have even argued that many people are experiencing *nature deficit disorder* (Louv, 2008) and *environmental generational amnesia* (Kahn et al., 2009) due to modern practices, which often detract from meaningful interactions with nature and animals. Importantly, both the concept of *nature deficit disorder* and *environmental generational amnesia* have been hypothesized to contribute to decreased physical health and well-being. In our book, we have considered how VHAIs might support – rather than detract from – a vital reconnection with nature and animals. For instance, many virtual human-animal connections include diverse animals (i.e., companion and wild or farm animals) and often situate animals within their natural habitats. Future empirical research could explore if VHAIs might serve a dual purpose, that is, foster people's reconnection with the natural world while simultaneously supporting their learning, social connections, and well-being. This is an interesting area for future study in the field of VHAIs.

Echoing calls from the broader field of mental health to offer culturally responsive and scalable mental health interventions that can be easily accessed by varied community members (Alvarez et al., 2022), what might culturally responsive VHAIs look like? How might the content of virtual interventions reflect both *content* and *approaches* that honour the cultural contexts and ways of knowing of different and varied viewers? In their systematic review of internet-delivered health interventions, Rogers and colleagues (2017) posit that such interventions are enhanced when accompanied by a corresponding website that can be accessed by viewers seeking additional or follow-up information. Future VHAIs could examine the effects of a comprehensive hybrid intervention comprised of a virtual AAI that sees participants not only synchronously participate in virtual sessions but also participate in asynchronous extension activities via a website showcasing information or activities germane to the virtual AAI itself.

In addition, as is the case within the broader field of HAIs, the field of VHAIs would be strengthened with the addition of qualitative research to capture subtle nuances in the experiences of all stakeholders including animals, handlers, and participants (Fournier, 2019; Kazdin, 2017; Kuzura et al., 2019; Shapiro, 2020). For instance, qualitative observations and/or case studies would speak to whether there are features of the animal, handler, or the handler-animal team that are more therapeutic or likely to support benefits for participants. Qualitative research would also allow for more detailed exploration of the links among participants' characteristics (e.g., age, previous experience with technology and interaction with animals) and their VHAI experiences. Moving forward, research is needed that explores: What factors make for a successful handler in a VHAI session? What dynamics characterize a successful dog-handler team in a VHAI session? What type of animal captures the attention of younger or older virtual audiences, and why? What are the best ways to engage virtual viewers across the lifespan and various backgrounds? For whom does a synchronous or asynchronous delivery of virtual human-animal interaction work best? Qualitative research can begin to address these exciting questions and, in doing so, will push forward the fields of HAIs and VHAIs.

Conclusion

The subfield of VHAIs, an emerging area of practice and study under the larger umbrellas of HAIs and AAIs, is an exciting and dynamic area of study. It is a field that harnesses technology and all its capabilities to create opportunities for humans to interact with animals in varied virtual contexts. As we bring our book to a close, we invite readers to put into practice the findings from studies reviewed throughout this book and to boldly advance the study and practice of virtual human-animal interactions.

References

Alvarez, J. C., Waitz-Kudla, S., Brydon, C., Crosby, E., & Witte, T. K. (2022). Culturally responsive scalable mental health interventions: A call to action. *American Psychological Association, 8*(3), 406–415. https://doi.org/10.1037/tps0000319.

Barker, S. B., Barker, R. T., McCain, N. L., & Schubert, C. M. (2016). A randomized cross-over exploratory study of the effect of visiting therapy dogs on college student stress before final exams. *Anthrozoös, 29*(1), 35–46. https://doi.org/10.1080/08927936.2015.1069988

Bekoff, M. (2014). *Rewilding our hearts: Building pathways of compassion and coexistence*. New World Library.

Bennet, B., & Woodman, E. (2019). The potential of equine-assisted psychotherapy for treating trauma in Australian Aboriginal peoples. *British Journal of Social Work, 49*, 1049–1058. https://doi.org/10.1093/bjsw/bcz053

Binfet, J. T., Green, F. L. L., & Draper, Z. A. (2022a). The importance of client-canine contact in canine-assisted interventions: A randomized controlled trial. *Anthrozoös, 35*(1), 1–22. https://doi.org/10.1080/08927936.2021.1944558

Binfet, J. T., Passmore, H. A., Cebry, A., Struik, K., & McKay, C. (2018). Reducing university students' stress through a drop-in canine-therapy program. *Journal of Mental Health, 27*(3), 197–204. https://doi.org/10.1080/09638237.2017.1417551

Binfet, J. T., Tardif-Williams, C. Y., Draper, Z. A., Green, F. L. L., Rousseau, C. X., & Roma, R. (2022b). Virtual canine comfort: A randomized controlled trial of the effects of a canine-assisted intervention supporting undergraduate well-being. *Anthrozoös, 35*(6), 809–832. https://doi.org/10.1080/08927936.2022.2062866

Dell, C., Williamson, L., McKenzie, H. Carey, B., Cruz, M., Gibson, M., & Pavelich, A. (2021). A commentary about lessons learned: Transitioning a therapy dog program online during the Covid-19 pandemic. *Animals, 11*, 914. https://doi.org/10.3390/ani11030914

Ein, N., Gervasio, J., Reed, M. J., & Vickers, K. (2022). Effects on wellbeing of exposure to dog videos before a stressor. *Anthrozoos*, 1–19. https://doi.org/10.1080/08927936.2022.2149925

Fournier, A. (2019). *Animal-assisted intervention*. Palgrave Macmillan.

Kahn, P. H., Severson, R. L., & Ruckert, J. H. (2009). The human relation with nature and technological nature. *Current Directions in Psychological Science, 18*(1), 37–42. https://doi.org/10.1111/j.1467-8721.2009.01602.x

Kazdin, A. E. (2017). Strategies to improve the evidence base of animal-assisted interventions. *Applied Developmental Science, 21*(2), 150–164. https://doi.org/10.1080/10888691.2016.1191952

Kuzara, S., Pendry, P., & Gee, N. R. (2019). Exploring the handler-dog connection within a university-based animal-assisted activity. *Animals, 9*(7), 402. http://dx.doi.org/10.3390/ani9070402

Louv, R. (2008). *Last child in the woods: Saving our children from nature-deficit disorder*. Algonquin Books of Chapel Hill.

Marcus, D. A. (2013). The science behind animal-assisted therapy. *Current Pain and Headache Reports, 17*, 322. https://doi.org/10.1007/s11916-013-0322-2

Nepps, P., Stewart, C. N., & Bruckno, S. R. (2014). Animal-assisted activity: Effects of a complementary intervention program on psychological and physiological variables. *Journal of Evidence-Based Complementary & Alternative Medicine, 19*, 211–215. https://doi.org/10.1177/2156587214533570

Nimer, J., & Lundahl, B. (2007). Animal-assisted therapy: A meta-analysis. *Anthrozoos, 20*, 225–238. https://doi.org/10.2752/089279307X224773

Pendry, P., Carr, A. M., Vandagriff, J. L., & Gee, N. R. (2021). Incorporating human-animal interaction into academic stress management programs: Effects on typical and at-risk college students' executive function. *AERA Open, 7*(1), 1–18. https://journals.sagepub.com/home/ero

Rogers, M. A. M., Lemmen, K., Kramer, R., Mann, J., & Chopra, V. (2017). Internet-delivered health interventions that work: Systematic review of meta-analyses and evaluation of website availability. *Journal of Medical Internet Research, 19*(3), e90. www.jmit.org/2017/e90/

Rossetti, J., & King, C. (2010). Use of animal-assisted therapy with psychiatric patients: A literature review. *Journal of Psychosocial Nursing and Mental Health Services, 48*(11), 44–48.

Rousseau, C. X., Binfet, J. T., Green, F. L. L., Tardif-Williams, C., Draper, Z., & Maynard, A. (2020). Up the leash: An investigation of handler well-being and perceptions of volunteering in canine-assisted interventions. *Pet Behavior Science, 10*, 15–35. https://doi.org/10.2107/pbs.vi10.12598I

Scheck, H., Williamson, L., & Dell, C. A. (2022). Understanding psychiatric patients' experiences of virtual animal-assisted therapy sessions during COVID-19 pandemic. *People and Animals: The International Journal of Research and Practice, 5*(1), Article 6. https://docs.lib.purdue.edu/paij/vol5/iss1/6

Shapiro, K. (2020). Human-animal studies: Remembering the past, celebrating the present, troubling the future. *Society and Animals, 28*(7), 797–833. https://doi.org/10.1163/15685306-bja10029

Steel, J. (2023). Reading to dogs in schools: A controlled feasibility study of an online Reading to Dogs intervention. *International Journal of Educational Research, 117*, 102117. https://doi.org/10.1016/j.ijer.2022.102117

Tardif-Williams, C. Y., Binfet, J. T., Green, F. L. L., Roma, R., Akshat, S., Rousseau, C. X., & Godard, R. J. (2023). When therapy dogs provide virtual comfort: Exploring university students' insights and perspectives. *People and Animals: The International Journal of Research and Practice, 6*(1), 1–17. https://docs.lib.purdue.edu/paij/vol6/iss1/5

Index

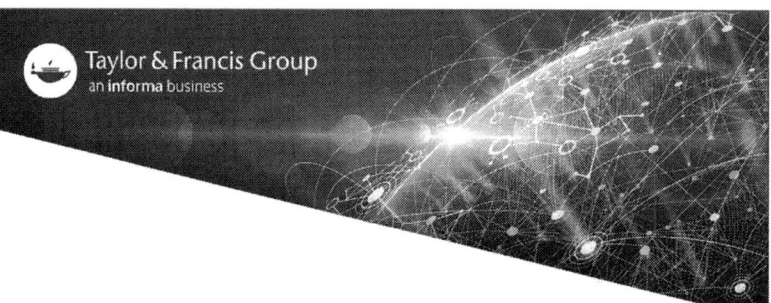
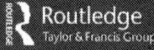
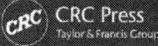